IMMIGRANT PHYSICIANS

*To Dr Watson
Best Wishes*

*Ghazi Rayan
8-22-2024*

To Dr Watson
Best wishes
Chris Hoefer
8-22-2024

Immigrant Physicians

Their Contributions and Influence
on American Medical History

Ghazi Rayan MD

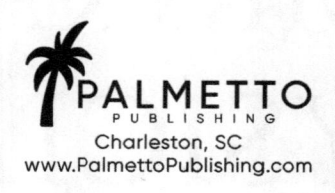

PALMETTO
PUBLISHING
Charleston, SC
www.PalmettoPublishing.com

Immigrant Physicians
Copyright © 2023 by Ghazi Rayan MD

All rights reserved

No portion of this book may be reproduced, stored in a retrieval system, or transmitted in any form by any means—electronic, mechanical, photocopy, recording, or other—except for brief quotations in printed reviews, without prior permission of the author.

Hardcover ISBN: 979-8-8229-1694-4
Paperback ISBN: 979-8-8229-1695-1
eBook ISBN: 979-8-8229-1696-8

Table of Contents

Preface — vii
Chapter 1: Evolution of Medicine — 1
Chapter 2: Anatomical Science and Anatomists — 36
Chapter 3: American Medical Education and Educators — 55
Chapter 4: Colonial and Revolutionary War Physicians — 70
Chapter 5: Civil War Physicians — 87
Chapter 6: Antebellum Physicians with Non-medical Contributions — 116
Chapter 7: Physicians at the Dawn of Modern Medicine — 126
Chapter 8: Physicians in Specialized Fields — 161
Chapter 9: Award-Winning Physicians — 194
Chapter 10: Women Physicians — 218
Chapter 11: American Healthcare — 238
Chapter 12: My Medical Journey — 261
Conclusion — 283
References — 289
List of Immigrant Physicians and Health Professionals — 300
Acknowledgments — 310
About the Author — 311

Preface

Since Europeans first landed on American shores some five hundred years ago and settled in the "New World," immigrants have flocked from every corner of the globe to this new land of opportunity. These newcomers helped found and foster the social fabric of the US; they transformed the vast barren terrains into sprawling cities, towns, and villages. During the Industrial Revolution, demand for labor attracted unschooled immigrant laborers, while the burgeoning technological revolution would create prospects for the highly skilled: engineers, inventors, intellectuals, scientists, thinkers, and physicians.

The population density of the new country swelled. During the 1700s, the English colonial population doubled almost every 25 years. With just 260,000 settlers in 1700, the population would increase eight times over to a total of 2,150,000 in the following 70 years and reaching 5,300,000 in 1800. By the turn of the 19th century, the two most populous cities were New York and Philadelphia, followed by Baltimore and Boston. The population of the New York urban area in 1800 was 60,000; by 1850, it was nearly 600,000. Philadelphia proper was second to New York City, with roughly 40,000 in 1800 and 120,000 50 years later.

This urbanization brought with it overcrowding, poor hygienic practices, and increased risk of the spread of infectious diseases. Let's take New York City as one example of these new urban communities. In the 1800s, sanitation was non-existent in New York City, and residents simply dumped their trash and waste on streets in anticipation of it being collected by scavengers. Norwegian rats that came on ships from England were the most prominent scavengers of this street trash, which became a convenient breeding ground for their own population explosion. After the rain, raw sewage from homes and waste from factories would drain into rivers and lakes, contaminating the city's water supply with microbes and chemicals. People became sick from drinking this unhealthy water; those who could afford to do so instead drank fermented and brewed beverages—like beer, ale, cider, and wine.

Horses were central to the smooth operation of the nineteenth-century city. They provided transportation for people and moved cargo from trains into the growing metropolis. By 1880, there were roughly 150,000 horses in the city; and of course, these horses ate and excreted. At a rate of 22 pounds per horse per day, their manure added up to millions of pounds a day and over 100,000 tons per year—in addition to around 10 million gallons of horse urine. Streets were literally carpeted and buried in a warm, brown foul-smelling thick stew of horse-human muck. When it rained, the streets would turn to a sludge; when the weather was hot and dry, the wind stirred up a toxic dust of manure particles. Dead horses littered the streets and were left to decompose, offering a sumptuous feast to billions of buzzing flies. The "great horse manure crisis of 1894" in London was present in almost every large US city. In fact, one of the greatest obstacles to urban development at the turn of the century was the difficulty in removing horse manure from the streets **(Fig 1)**. Affluent brownstone homes in Baltimore and

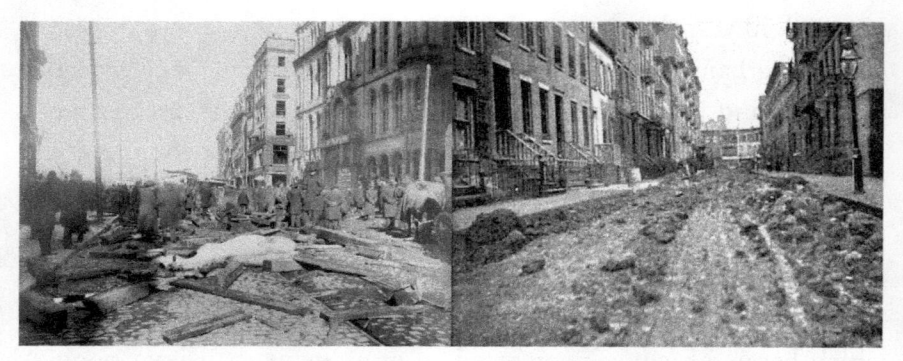

Fig 1. New York City during the 1890s' "Horse Manure Crisis". Dead horses, horse manure and dumped trash carpeted city streets, instigating health hazards and obstacles to urban development. (99% Invisible)

Brooklyn were built high with front doors accessed by several stone or marble stoops to avoid the grime of the streets.

As elsewhere in the country, health conditions in New York by the mid-1800s had deteriorated drastically. Cholera and scarlet fever came in waves; malaria and tuberculosis were rampant. Epidemics plagued the lives of many New Yorkers in the form of smallpox, typhus, yellow fever, measles, malaria, and—in 1900—the plague. Deadly waves of cholera swept through New York in 1832, 1849, and 1866, killing thousands of people and infecting thousands more. During the cholera years, mortality rates soared to heights almost double those at the beginning of the century and killed approximately 1 in 20 residents. Scarlet fever and measles, on average, claimed the lives of 100 to 200 children during non-epidemic years and far greater numbers during outbreaks.

In those days, physicians and surgeons had their work cut out for them, whether in times of peace, war, or epidemics. During the Revolutionary War, men sustained a variety of wounds produced by low-velocity weapons: musket balls, bayonets, swords, arrows, and tomahawks. Crushing injuries often occurred from overturned wagons or fallen horses. To treat their injuries, there were about 3,500 practicing physicians in the colonies in 1775. While these doctors were well-trained by the standards of their time, their services were in short supply to the vast population of sick and wounded soldiers.

Army surgeons during the Civil War were committed to care for massive war casualties, and the innumerable survivors of those conflicts in the following decades. In the 1800s, most doctors traveled by foot or horseback to wealthy patients' homes. Patients, who could not afford visits to their homes, went to the hospital for treatment where they more often died than were cured. On the eve of the Civil War, there were 40,000 practicing physicians in the country—plus, over 16,000 pseudo physicians, who were barely trained and practiced in non-official capacities. Most legitimate physicians of the antebellum period were trained through apprenticeships; some attended the few medical schools, which had established themselves. To enhance their knowledge, physicians who could afford to travel sought further training in Europe, where medicine was more advanced and medical schools abounded. Immigrant physicians who came to America from Europe around the Revolutionary and Civil War periods had attended European medical schools and were proficiently trained. They were a blessing to a growing country desperately in need of medical expertise. There is no demographic information as to the ratio of immigrant to American born physicians from that era.

As an immigrant American, I have often mused upon these questions: How many American immigrants have made critical contributions to this nation's institutions and constitution? What notions and initiatives did they offer that favorably impacted the course of this country's history? To seek answers to these nagging questions, I searched the literature to discover that the number of immigrants arriving on American shores who enacted transformative change is simply staggering. I amassed a myriad of names and entries on immigrants whose accomplishments span the full spectrum of disciplines: architecture, business, economy, education, environment, journalism, literature, medicine, visual arts, and many more.

This compelled me to write the book Immigrants *Who Founded and Fostered an Early Nation* (2021). In that first volume, I narrowed my historical focus to cover the early migrations, explorers, settlers, slave trade, immigration laws, and ethnic immigration. The book also profiled over 200 immigrants who made exemplary political contributions to their newfound home, including the founding fathers, framers of the Constitution, war heroes and heroines, justices, and financers.

My investigation culminated with an overview of the many immigrant American physicians whose inspiring stories are now more expansively covered in the pages of the book you are reading. Those Immigrant physicians throughout American history provided a necessary health care to their patients, enhancing the wellbeing of countless communities. Some served as army surgeons in the Revolutionary War or oversaw conflicts that helped win the nation's independence. Others served in the Civil War—mostly in the Union Army—and helped save the Union. Those who served on the Confederate side also cared for injured soldiers during and after the war. Immigrant physicians also, throughout the 19th and 20th centuries, were responsible for important therapeutic discoveries, medical innovations and health programs that laid the foundations of the modern American medical care system we all enjoy today.

Our knowledge of this past history is, of course, necessarily partial. It is but a fragment of the myriad stories lucky enough to be set to paper. Historical knowledge can be all too easily lost, as would be the case in the great fire at the ancient Library of Alexandria where countless records of the Ancient Egyptians and Sumerians were lost. We may not know how many immigrant physicians crossed the Atlantic and contributed to unchronicled medical advances. We only know of those that were recorded. Therefore, included within the pages of this book you will find only the accounts of those immigrants whose momentous medical breakthroughs were documented. The profiles of these extraordinary immigrant physicians, men and women, past and not present, to tell their own tale, somehow express something timeless and transcendental about the human condition and our instinct to help the unknown other.

This book is also a voyage of discovery of the early history of Medicine and its practices and ailments. Exploring the lives, the stories, and the times of those physicians helps us to understand our own narrative; it helps us appreciate the true values of the promise of medical privilege that we enjoy and so often take for granted; it helps us embrace diversity and know what it means to be an American.

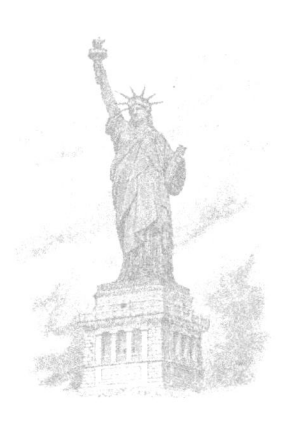

CHAPTER 1

Evolution of Medicine

Medicine evolved over millennia and became enriched by a succession of civilizations from Mesopotamia, ancient Egypt, China and India to ancient Greece, Rome and the European empires. Greco-Roman physicians and those of the Islamic Golden Age propagated their remedial knowledge to clinicians of the Renascence and Enlightenment. Medical practices were refined and delivered by Europeans to practitioners of the colonies. And so it was, the foundation of modern American medicine was built on scientific innovations engendered by formative, thoughtful inventors and researchers. These technological breakthroughs cured diseases, controlled epidemics, prolonged people's lifespan and improved their quality of life. This chapter will delve into the history and dynamics that shaped medicine that we know today.

Medicine Through the Ages and Civilizations

The history of Medicine is the history of Civilization itself. For many anthropologists, Civilization can be traced back to our first evidence of one human nursing another back to good health: In the animal kingdom, a broken limb is a death sentence for any member of a group of hunter-gatherers; however, Margaret Mead famously suggested that a first human skeleton found buried alongside others with a fractured femur which healed was the first evidence we have of humankind nurturing others back to good health before resuming their nomadic existence.

Medicine is an epic odyssey stretching back into the depths of the prehistoric Stone Age, which ended 35,000 BCE. Mesopotamia, an area in the Middle East, witnessed not only the first, but a succession of civilizations. Its first empire, the Sumerians, arose around 4500 BCE and was conquered by the Akkadian Empire around 2270 BCE. Besides inventing the wheel, the city, and laws (known as the Hammurabi codes), the Sumerians also developed the first known systems of writing—on clays and stone tablets—around 3400 BCE. The number of clay tablets recovered today exceeds 500,000. These were written upon by Sumerians and later Babylonians, Akkadians, Assyrians, and Hittites. The British Museum contains the largest collection outside of Iraq; approximately 130,000 texts and fragments. The oldest is the Sumerian Epic of Gilgamesh, which dates from 2100 BCE. Medicine in Mesopotamia was already practiced by the time of the Babylonian and Assyrian eras. Sumerian medical clay tablets were discovered from about 3,000 BCE and are considered the oldest known medical writings. Similar tablets were also found from Babylonia **(Fig 2)**.

The ancient Egyptian civilization followed soon after, initially coalescing around 3100 BCE; it would last a total of 3000 years. Ancient Egypt is considered the cradle of Modern Medicine where detailed treatments were written on papyrus, an early form of paper. Ancient Egyptian medicine was one of the earliest reported professional practices. Egyptians would go on to influence Greek physicians; many of whom visited Egypt. Toward the end of the Egyptian dynasties, when Egypt fell to the Roman Empire, Alexandria became a medical center that attracted physicians from many parts of the world. The Library of

Alexandria was the center of all scientific and medical knowledge.

The Indus, the first civilization of the Indian subcontinent, would come into existence around 2500 BCE. Their ancient medical science, known as *Ayurveda*, was a healing method that relied on herbs for maintaining good health. It was practiced by sages who continue to use its central techniques of meditation, massage, yoga, laxatives, and enemas. There is some debate as to whether civilization would emerge in China before or after India, but it is likely both emerged more or less simultaneously and coexisted. Xia, the earliest dynasty, appeared around 2070 BCE and China can consequently claim the longest continuous history of any civilization—spanning a total of 3500 years. Chinese traditional medicine has used herbs and acupuncture since 1050 BCE.

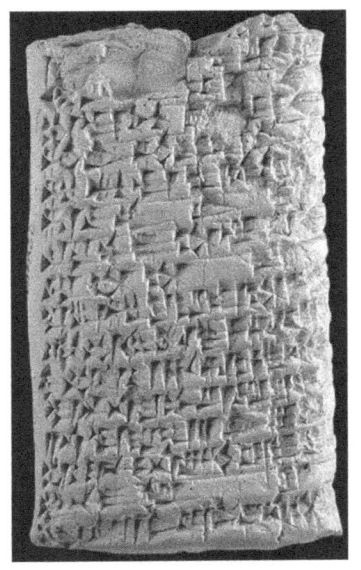

Fig 2. Medical clay tablet from Old Babylonia Period (1792–1595 BCE) with incantation against several diseases. (Spurlock Museum of World Cultures)

Europeans would soon begin to follow this trend. The Greek Civilization began around 800 BCE, declining with the death of Alexander the Great and ending around 30 BCE when they were defeated by the Romans. Greeks achieved medical milestones through the use of logic and would change the trajectory of medicine forever, laying the foundations of the medical practice that followed. Greek medicine was the outcome of Hippocrates' teachings and a quintessential dynamism that changed the way physicians practiced their profession at that time. Hippocrates visited Egypt, where he studied medicine before returning to Greece. The Greek medicine of Hippocrates, albeit rooted in the 'four humors', also ushered in the altruistic and ethical practice of medicine.

The two enduring contributions of the Greeks to modern medicine are the 'Caduceus staff' and the Hippocratic oath. The 'Caduceus staff' of the Greek messenger god, Hermes, has become a symbol for medicine: it features two snakes winding up around the length of a staff topped with wings. Although the symbol may have first appeared in Mesopotamia, it is derived from Asclepius, Greek god of medicine and healing, who could supposedly bring people from the dead. His staff is portrayed as a single rod with one winding snake. Ancient Greeks visited temples to implore Asclepius for cure from disease. In 1902, US army medical corps adopted Caduceus as a logo. Many medical organizations today use the symbol as their emblem, including the US Public Health Service.

As Romans conquered most of the civilized world, the Golden Age of Greece and its medicine ended. The Roman Empire itself lasted nearly 1000 years; it was founded in 625 BCE and ended in 476 CE. Rome was established earlier in 753 BCE, and Augustus Caesar proclaimed himself its first emperor in 31 BCE. The fall of Rome began in 410 CE when the Barbarians invaded it. Medicine during the Roman Empire was greatly influenced by the Greeks and many physicians came from Greece to spread their knowledge in Rome. Romans did not allow the dissection of corpses, which hindered the advancement of anatomy and medicine. They did, however, adopt the cult of Aesculapius, and even built shrines for him, particularly at spas and thermal baths, which would have their own in-house doctors.

Roman medicine was disseminated by Greek physicians who improved its practice through the study of animal anatomy and (illegal) human dissection. One of the leading proponents of anatomy was the Greek Galen who learned from examining the wounds of injured gladiators and studying cadavers, carefully circumventing the harsh laws against dissecting human bodies. One of the greatest tragedies of that time was the burning of the Alexandria library in 48 BCE along with

40,000 to 400,000 scrolls, which had been gathered and preserved over hundreds of years.

The Middle Ages was the subsequent period in European history that followed the collapse of the Roman Empire and lasted until the Renaissance, extending from 500 through 1400 CE. The collapse of the Roman Empire was triggered when the Vandals began to ransack Rome in 400 CE ushering in a new dark era in Europe. The early Middle Ages was dubbed the 'Dark Ages' by Petrarch because there was a notable lack of scientific and cultural advancements. That period also witnessed economic and cultural decline. Religious influence came to dominate all else, and the Roman Catholic Church considered illness a punishment from God—so those who fell ill were considered sinners. This period also witnessed the rise of Islam, the Crusades, rise of Catholic Church and Spain, population expansion, building of universities and London and Paris being the largest of cities.

In the early Middle Ages, the practice of medicine continued to be rooted in Greek traditions with Arabic and Jewish doctors often employed by kings. Medicine during the Dark Ages experienced a significant decline, however, due to famine, wars, and epidemics such as Bubonic plague, which swept across Europe. To cure disease, wise men and women used magic stones and practiced witchcraft, apothecaries used herbal elixirs, and priests used prayers. Barbers acted as surgeons and used crude methods of treatment; even physicians employed cruel practices such as bloodletting to treat many ailments, a practice that lasted for centuries. Many of the previous gains made in the medical field by the Greeks, Romans, and Muslims were abandoned and forgotten. However, some advances were destined to emerge later in that era; these included a proliferation of universities and the invention of surgical devices by Muslim physicians. By the twelfth century, medical schools had been established throughout Europe. The Medical School of Salerno in Italy was founded by a Christian, an Arab, and a Jew.

In the Late Middle Ages, Physicians adopted the art of diagnosis and began to use opiates for surgery. Barber surgeons began to thrive as a profession, and physicians made some small progress in adopting new treatments and surgical methods. Hospitals, such as Saint Bartholomew in London and the Hotel Dieu in Paris, began to emerge but were far from the hospitals of today.

It's difficult to say exactly where the Middle Ages end and the Renaissance begin. Ultimately, a new era dawned at different moments in different corners of Europe. The 'Renaissance' itself means 'rebirth' and is generally described as the period lasting from the beginning of the 14th century to the beginning of the 17th century. It commenced in Italy but was an important phase in European history as it led to a huge advance in many disciplines including art, literature, philosophy, music, science, and medicine. It was the bridge that connected the Middle Ages with modern times. It was also a period of renewed interest in old knowledge. Greek, Arabic, and Persian medical texts were translated into Latin. The availability of Gutenberg's printing press from 1440 onwards allowed the rapid spread of medical textbooks. As the Church's influence receded, greater medical experiments were undertaken, and many new discoveries took place. Novel treatments were introduced, such as vaccinations, which helped curb epidemics. The Scientific Revolution began in earnest, however, toward the end of the Renascence.

The 17th and 18th centuries were considered the Age of Enlightenment in Europe, but in America, they were the Age of Colonialism where medicine lagged behind the Europeans. Religious hierarchies and social constraints were rejected by Enlightenment thinkers in favor of new freedoms. The 18th century in Europe is viewed as a critical period in the history of medicine, as populations became the subject of large-scale interventions in response to epidemics and mass inoculation programs. Public Health and Hygiene began receiving serious attention. The age of modern medicine truly began in the mid 18th century, which coincided with the Industrial Revolution in Western Europe and America. It witnessed an expansion in medical science that contributed to the prevention and cure of many diseases and increased the longevity and wellbeing of many people's lives. This era witnessed the development of new methods and approaches for examining the body and the emergence of new ideas about how the body functions. Medicine became professionalized, and ordinary people adopted a more optimistic outlook on the role and benefits of medicine.

During the early part of the 19th century, some medical practices continued to rely on symptomatic treatment, consisting primarily of bloodletting, blistering, and high doses of mineral poisons. A few medical practitioners still believed in the ancient creed of the "four humors." However, as the 1800s drew to a close, physicians began applying much smaller doses of effective medicines and some major discoveries took place. It was a time of exponential growth for medicine in Europe where discoveries multiplied, and countless eminent physicians introduced new ideas that would set the stage for modern medicine.

Thanks to many immigrant-physicians from Europe, American medicine in the late 19th century and early 20th centuries began to rival European medicine. The 19th century's most momentous discoveries emerged in 1846, 1865, and 1895—and they would change the face of medicine forever. These innovations are x-rays, anesthesia, antisepsis, and antibiotics.

Ancient and Early Physicians

The first physician ever known to man was from ancient Egypt. Two foremost physicians of ancient Greece demystified and dispelled old dogmas about the source of disease and how the body functions. But it was scores of Medieval Islamic clinicians who advanced the fields of medicine and surgery where some of their ideas are being implemented today.

Imhotep (2667-2600 BCE), the earliest known non-royal Egyptian physician in history, was one of Pharaoh Djoser's chief chancellors during the third dynasty of the Old Kingdom. He was also an astronomer, astrologist, politician, and architect, credited with building the first stepped pyramid in Saqqara. After his death, Imhotep was deified as God of healing and medicine. He is sometimes illustrated in figurines as holding a cup of medicine. More than four thousand years later in 1862, Edwin Smith, an American collector of antiquities, found and purchased a papyrus manuscript that became known as the Edwin Smith surgical papyrus. This is the world's oldest surgical text on trauma and was translated in 1930, though it dates back to about 1600 BCE to unknown scribe. It is a scroll 15.3 feet long written in hieroglyphics and describes the work of Imhotep **(Fig 3)**. The 48 cases detailed injuries, wounds, fractures, and dislocations. Fractured hands and skulls were included along with skin abscesses. It also described eight cases of breast tumors with a vivid account of breast cancer.

Hippocrates of Cos (460 BCE -370 BCE) is dubbed as the "Father of Modern Medicine". He was a Greek physician who dismissed supernatural sources of disease but considered human body to have four cardinal fluids or 'humors': blood, black bile, yellow bile, and phlegm, all of which coexisted in perfect balance. Disease, he declared, is caused by

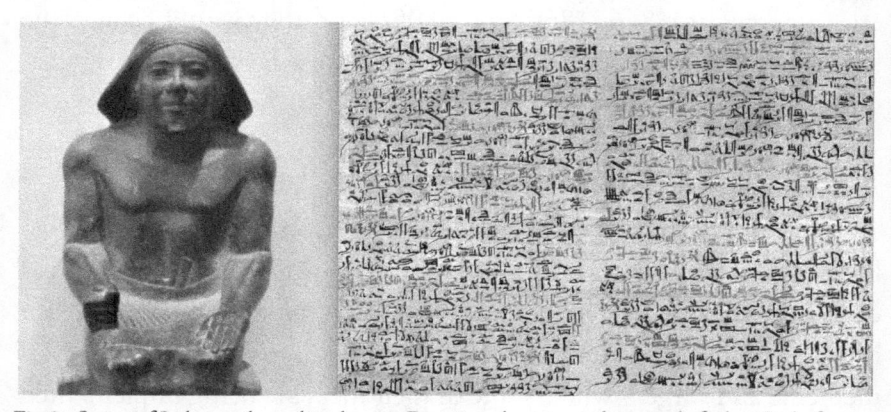

Fig 3. Statue of Imhotep the earliest known Egyptian physician in history, deified as God of healing and medicine, his hieroglyphic surgical papyrus was discovered by Edwin Smith. (Cairo Museum 2018)

an imbalance of these humors. The Hippocratic Corpus is a collection of about 60 Ancient Greek medical texts attributed to Hippocrates, and his teachings discussed medical theories, illnesses, and the ethics of medical practice. The corpus became the foundation of the Western medical tradition. In his time, the word for cancer, *karkinos*, first appeared in the medical literature and the tumor was portrayed by Hippocrates as a crab buried in the sand with limbs spread in a circle. Hippocrates also wrote the Hippocratic oath for physicians to swear to practice medicine ethically. Modernized versions of the code of medical ethics are still used today.

Other prominent Greek physicians and anatomists include Herophilos (335–280 BCE) and Galen of Pergamon (129–216 BCE), who lived during the Roman Empire and who made substantial contributions to physiology, pathology, pharmacology, and neurology (anatomy chapter).

Fortunately, Romans decided to build on Greek medicine. Some Roman physicians also made contributions to medicine, though many were Greeks living in the Roman Empire who had studied in Alexandria. Soranus of Ephesus (98-138 BCE) is best known for his remarkable work, *On Midwifery and the Diseases of Women*. Aulus Celsus (25 BCE – 50 CE) published *De Medicina*, a text on diet, pharmacy, and surgery, which is the only surviving section of a much larger encyclopedia. Oribasius (320 – 403 CE) acted as personal physician to the Roman emperor Julian and wrote the *Medical Collections*, a massive compilation of excerpts from other medical writers from around the ancient world.

Medieval Islamic clinicians popularized Greco-Roman ideas and made sizeable contributions of their own that advanced the fields of medicine and surgery. They translated Greek works into Arabic, and many of their own works were later translated into Latin. Countless pioneer Muslim physicians spread knowledge from Iraq and Syria to Spain and beyond. The contributions of Muslim physicians and surgeons were undeniably superior to those that came before them and lasted much longer than those that came after them. They were responsible for what became known as the Islamic Golden Age. There are many individuals worth mentioning; only a few will be highlighted here, though.

Al Zahrawi (936–1013), whose principal work is the *Kitab al-Tasrif*, a thirty-volume encyclopedia of medical practices. The surgery segment attained great popularity and became the standard textbook in Europe for 500 years. He designed more than 200 surgical instruments, some of which are still used today. He pioneered the use of catgut sutures for repairing wounds. He was the first physician to identify the hereditary nature of hemophilia, describe ectopic abdominal pregnancy, and develop surgical devices for Caesarean sections and cataract surgeries.

Al-Razi (865-925), also known in the Western world as 'Rhazes', was one of the greatest physicians of the medieval period and was born in Persia. He wrote 200 books on alchemy, medicine, and philosophy—as well as the first book on pediatrics. He discussed the importance of medical ethics in service of the whole human race, where physicians should treat even their enemies. He contradicted some of Galen's teachings. His groundbreaking book titled, after translation, *Book of Medicine* (900 CE), was written after his death by his students and inspired many physicians in Europe and Islamic world.

Abu Ali Ibn Sina, (980 – 1037 CE), also known as Avicenna, was a Persian polymath, who is regarded as one of the most significant physicians, astronomers, and philosophers of the Islamic Golden Age. He preserved medical practices of Greece and Rome. Two hundred forty of his books survive to this day, of which 40 were on medicine, with his most influential publications being *The Book of Healing* and the five-book medical encyclopedia *al-Qanun fi al-tibb* (1025), also known as *The Cannon of Medicine*—which was originally written in Arabic **(Fig 4)**. The book covered many topics with great detail and precision. It discussed cancer surgery, infections such as tuberculosis,

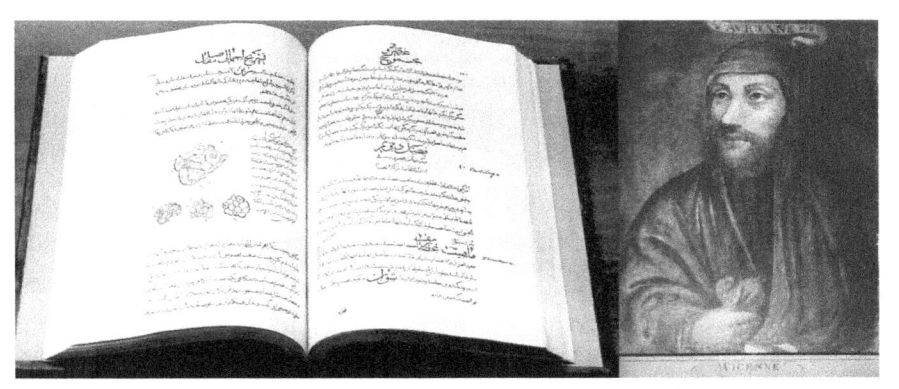

Fig 4. Avicenna Persian polymath, one of the most renowned physicians of the Islamic Golden Age, his textbook "The Cannon of Medicine" was written in Arabic. (Wikimedia/Wikipedia)

and psychiatric disorders such as hallucinations and depression. He advocated for proper drug testing and clinical trials on multiple patients. The book remained a key text in universities for over 500 years. Johns Hopkins physician William Osler wrote of Avicenna that he was the "author of the most famous medical textbook ever written" and his Cannon was described as providing "a medical bible for a longer time than any other work."

Ibn Zuhr, (1094–1162) is known for his emphasis on the rational, empiric basis of medicine. Several of his major discoveries were chronicled in his book on therapeutics and diet and another on psychology. He performed the first-ever experimental tracheotomy on a goat.

Al-Nafis (1213-1288) was an Arab anatomist, physician, and polymath, born in Syria and working in Egypt. He wrote an encyclopedia of 80 volumes entitled *The Comprehensive Book on Medicine*, which is one of the largest medical compendiums ever written by one person. He was the first to describe the passage of blood between heart and lungs for oxygenation. For that, he was designated as "the father of circulatory physiology."

Jewish Physicians were also renowned for their knowledge of medicine alongside their Muslim counterparts. No medicine can be said to be distinctly Jewish, but rather ancient Jewish practitioners adopted both Greek and Greco-Roman medical knowledge. *The Book of Remedies*, the earliest medical text, was written in Hebrew by Asaph the Jew; it dates back to the 7th or 8th century. Not much is known about the author, but the book comprises four sections: a story of the transmission of medicine from God to mankind, a medical survey, description of different medicines, and a list of medical sayings. Judah Halevi (1075–1141) was a Spanish Jewish physician, poet, and philosopher. He was known as an accomplished physician, but more for his poetry, which was written in Arabic. He traveled to Jerusalem during the Crusades, where he died.

Maimonides (1138–1204), was a preeminent medieval Jewish philosopher, astronomer, and physician who was born in Córdoba. He practiced medicine in both Morocco and Egypt. He was one of the most prolific and influential Torah scholars of the Middle Ages and an authority on Jewish law and ethics. He received medical training in Córdoba and in Fez and gained a widespread reputation as a physician. He was appointed court physician to Sultan Saladin. Maimonides described conditions such as asthma, diabetes, hepatitis, and pneumonia, and his essays became influential for later physicians. He studied Greek and Arabic medicine and followed the principles of Galen but used his own experience to treat patients in a more personal manner. He died in Egypt but was buried in the Tiberias in Israel.

And so it was, on the shoulder of giants, that medical knowledge was passed from Greeks to Romans, from Romans to Muslims, from Muslims to medieval physicians, and onwards to the physicians of modern medicine.

Early Medical Practices

Witch doctors and medicine men have existed for thousands of years amongst tribal societies in Africa and the Americas, where sickness was attributed to supernatural powers. These practitioners performed ceremonies to communicate with the spirits and gave charms and plant-based treatments to the sick. They were feared and perceived as possessing powers to both hurt and heal, to kill and cure.

A combination of archaeological and anthropological studies showed that trepanation was the oldest operation ever performed, for which evidence exists in prehistoric human remains from 10,000 years ago. More than 1500-trephined skulls from the Neolithic period have been excavated globally. Surgical trepanation was conducted in prehistoric Africa and Europe, later becoming common in Mesoamerica and China. This process was executed by creating a hole in the human skull and removing a segment of the cranium. Its precise purpose remains unknown but it may have been intended to cure chronic disease: perhaps migraines or epilepsy. Unearthed skulls show healed bone margins, suggesting many survived the procedure. The Islamic al-Zahrāwī described in great detail how to perform the procedure with specific instruments.

Physicians in Mesopotamia used religious and ritual methods of treatment but also employed pharmaceutical, medical, and surgical means to treat patients. Mummified bodies, skeletal remains, wall paintings, and papyri have revealed that certain treatments also took place in ancient Egypt. Elaborate surgical instruments were seen engraved in a panel in Kom Ombo Temple, which include knives, hooks, shears, drills, saws, and forceps.

The practice of male circumcision originated in ancient Egypt long before Jewish and Muslim children were subjected to the procedure. On the door to the tomb of Pharaoh Ankhmahor, an engraving shows a priest performing circumcision on a boy around 2500 BCE, which is the oldest existing depiction of this operation. Circumcision was also used by South Sea Islanders, Aboriginal Australians, Sumatrans, Incas, Aztecs, and Mayans. Those societies implemented circumcision as ritual mutilation to test man's bravery and endurance, a sacrificial spilling of blood. Ensuing cultures used it as an initiation rite for manhood. Circumcision was even widely used by the British Army during WWII to prevent those serving in Asia and Africa from contracting sexually transmitted diseases. Recent studies conducted in Africa have shown that circumcision does lower the risk of contracting human immunodeficiency virus (HIV). Other health benefits of circumcision are improved local hygiene and a decreased risk of urinary tract infections and penile cancer.

After trepanation, limb amputation was the second most widely performed procedure in historic times. Bones from Egyptian dynasty were found dating to 2100 BCE with amputation and fusion of both bones of the forearm. An Egyptian mummy was discovered from 2400 years ago to have an artificial wood big toe and flexible leather, replacing an amputated toe that was still attached to the mummified remaining part of the foot; it is considered the earliest prosthesis. Findings also confirmed that ancient Egyptians treated fractures with wooden or bamboo splints especially for the forearm.

Traditional Chinese Medicine employed pressure, heat, and acupuncture to reach an equilibrium between the forces of *yin* and *yang*. The practice of acupuncture, where needles are inserted into specific points of the body, was first described as a system of diagnosis and treatment in *The Yellow Emperor's Classic of Internal Medicine*, which dates to 100 BCE. However, the basis of modern acupuncture was recorded in the Chinese *Great Compendium of Acupuncture and Moxibustion*, written during the Ming Dynasty by physician Yang Jizhou (1601). Although acupuncture today can be effective in relieving pain, some investigators believe it is achieved through the placebo effect.

Bloodletting is an ancient practice of bleeding a person, mainly through a vein, but sometimes an artery, in the arm using a lancet or knife. The intention was to rid the body of 'bad blood' or 'impure fluid,' and it was considered a cure for all ailments. It had its foundations in the observation of menstruation and was employed for thousands of years by Mesopotamians, Ancient Egyptians, Greeks, Romans, Aztecs, and Mayans. Galen advocated bleeding from the vein behind the ear to cure vertigo and headaches, whereas bloodletting from the temple was advocated to treat eye conditions. Bloodletting continued to be used throughout Medieval Europe and persisted as a common therapeutic method to treat diseases from gout to gonorrhea; in late 19th century, however, it began to fall out of fashion.

Barbershops today are still often best identified by a pole outside with red and white spiral stripes, though these originally referred to the blood and bandages that were the trappings of the barber-surgeon. Besides cutting hair, barbers in the 11th century performed bloodletting—among other procedures, such as extracting teeth and removing tumors with rusty knives. They performed bloodletting by tightly clutching the client's hand to engorge arm veins and then cutting to allow bleeding into a cup. The practice was widespread amongst all social classes: For example, King Charles II of England suffered seizures and was treated with bloodletting. President George Washington developed a terrible fever and respiratory problems after three physicians drew copious amounts of blood from him—he died the next day. Benjamin Rush was an ardent proponent of 'depletion therapy' and attempted to treat patients with yellow fever through bloodletting. Today, bloodletting or phlebotomy is still used to treat some blood diseases, such as hemochromatosis and polycythemia.

Less invasive but more ghastly methods of bloodletting is drawing blood from the body using live leaches. Leech therapy has been utilized for thousands of years to restore fluid balance. Despite lack of its favorable response, in the 18th-Century, leech madness hit Europe for treating almost any disease including mental illness. In some cases, dozens of leeches were applied to a person. The early barber pole was topped with a basin, representing container of leeches because they also utilized them. Leech therapy has made a comeback recently in microsurgery where it is employed for certain skin flaps and re-implanted amputated digits to alleviate venous congestion, thus preventing tissue death. A leech has three jaws with rows of small teeth, which pierce a person's skin producing anticoagulant enzymes allowing the parasitic worm absorbs congested blood. The live leech is allowed to extract blood, for 30 to 45 minutes at a time, which equates to about 5-10 ml of blood per leech each feeding; that is ten times its weight. However, because concerns about possible infections from these parasites, a "mechanical leech" has been developed recently.

The use of maggots to treat open wounds may seem repulsive, but it can be a life or limb-saving technique. Open wounds that lack sufficient blood supply can become a breeding ground for bacterial growth, causing septicemia and death. Maggots of the green bottle fly (Lucilia sericata) are able to secrete enzymes that liquefy dead tissue, leaving healthy tissue behind. Although patients may experience itching and squirming from hundreds of yellow-white swarming parasites on the wound, the use of maggots for wound treatment dates back centuries and has been scientifically proven to be effective. In fact, maggots have been used as a medical treatment since the American Civil War, when Confederate surgeon John Zacharias employed them to prevent septicemia and save hundreds of lives.

The trend for surgical debridement with a scalpel was initially preferred over maggot therapy, but this has changed in recent years. In the 1920s, an injured soldier was left on the battlefield for days and was found to have thousands of maggots on his wounds when he was brought to the hospital. The patient had no fevers, and his wounds were healing well. American orthopedic surgeon, William Baer, began using maggot therapy for chronic osteomyelitis in 1929, and he found that maggots were effective in debriding dead tissue, controlling infection, and allowing rapid healing. Studies have proven the efficacy of maggots, and they have been shown to be faster and more effective in cleaning dead tissue and forming healthy tissue compared to hydrogel dressings. Today, maggot therapy is approved for clinical use, and it is ideal for developing countries with limited resources.

In the Middle Ages, other bizarre remedies were used in Europe, including the use of urine as an antiseptic, cauterization with hot irons, and swallowing lead bullets for abdominal pain. In colonial America, hot irons were also used for cauterization, which caused further tissue damage and resulted in scar contracture and subsequent deformities. Meanwhile, John Brinkley, a quack from Kansas with no formal medical education, implanted goat testicles in men to cure male impotence. Although his license was eventually revoked in 1930, after twenty years of practice, he became wealthy with hundreds of thousands of followers and even ran for Kansas governor.

Early Ambulances and Hospitals

Transporting the sick or wounded to an infirmary has long featured as a priority throughout human history. The narrative of ambulances and hospitals began in ancient times. One primitive early example of an ambulance was invented by the Normans, who in the 11th century used a litter suspended between horses on two poles to transport the sick and injured. In 1487, Queen Isabella I, of Spain approved the construction of bedded wagons—a variation on the Norman litter—to carry wounded soldiers from battle to hospital tents, thus designing the earliest documented ambulance system.

A major shift in using battlefield ambulances began with the Frenchman Dominique Larrey, Napoleon Bonaparte's chief physician. Larrey rejected the Norman system of horse litters and instead developed covered, two- and four-wheeled horse-drawn wagons that could hold two or four fallen soldiers **(Fig 5)**. He later adapted his model for different circumstances, for Napoleon's army, using litter carried by a camel during the French campaign in Egypt (1798-1801). Civilian ambulances were first documented as transport carriages during the London cholera epidemic of 1832, which claimed 4000–7000 victims.

During the American Civil War, a Scottish-American immigrant **Alexander Skene** served as an assistant surgeon in the Union Army stationed in South Carolina and New York, and helped to create an army ambulance corp. At least one horse-drawn, two-wheeled ambulance

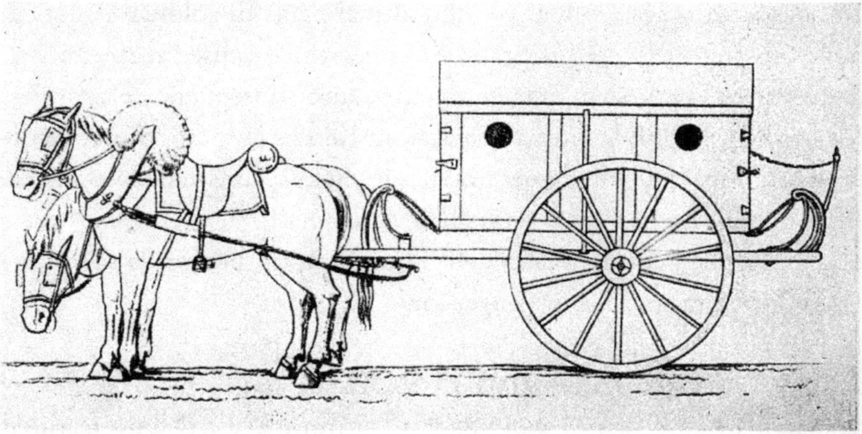

Fig 5. An early two-wheeled horse-drawn ambulance used by Dominique Larrey, Napoleon Bonaparte's chief physician. (Wikipedia)

cart was designated for each regiment, based on Larrey's model. These were often driven by volunteer civilians and carried equipment such as splints, morphine, and brandy. Steamboats and railroads were used for mass casualties after battles. In 1899, Michael Reese Hospital in Chicago was the first US institution to implement a motor-powered ambulance service, using an electric vehicle that ran on a 44-cell battery.

Hospitals have an equally extensive history to the ambulance. In ancient Egypt and Greece, temples functioned as centers for medical advice and healing. Historically, there was a connection between health and religion. Hospitals were funded by religious institutions and intended not only to save lives but souls. The end of the 4th century witnessed the founding of the first Christian hospital in the eastern Byzantine Empire by Saint Basil of Caesarea.

The Muslim world provides us with some of the first formal examples of multi-purpose hospitals, however. Persia hosted the Gundeshapur academy, which was founded in the 3rd century CE as an intellectual complex that contained a hospital, medical center, library, and observatory. Medieval Islamic hospitals were asylums for leprosy and blind patients, who were given stipends to support their families. The earliest Islamic general hospital was built in 805 in Baghdad by Harun Al-Rashid; by the 10th century, Baghdad had five more hospitals. The US National Library of Medicine credits the hospital as a product of medieval Islamic civilization.

During the Crusades of the 11th and 12th centuries, the "Order of Knights of the Hospital of Saint John of Jerusalem" set up hospitals to treat pilgrims wounded in battles for the "Holy Land", although there is no clear evidence as to how the wounded were transported to these hospitals.

In 1679, Louis XIV of France built a hospital and home for the elderly and sick children, which included a church. In 1784, Vienna General Hospital became the largest hospital encompassing 2000 beds and divided into wards for medicine surgery, venereal disease, a tower for the insane and a section for abandoned children. In 1736, Bellevue Hospital in New York City was founded as the oldest public hospital in the US.

Early Medicines

Medicines have accompanied Humankind throughout our existence. This section depicts where the foundation of Botany was laid and how myriad herbs were used as medicinal plants. We will see how the Ancient Egyptians and Chinese offered important early examples of such medicines, which would later be complemented by drugs like cocaine, opiates, aspirin, and other pharmaceuticals. So-called 'snake oil' salesmen have existed for just as long, however, so an important point of note is the advent of medicine patents and the efforts of people like Samuel Adams and Morris Fishbein to expose the dangers of fraudulent medicines.

In a burial site where a Neanderthal man was unearthed in 1960, eight species of plants were found, some of which are still being used for medicinal purposes. Ancient Egyptians in 3500 BCE and Chinese in 2700 BCE used herbs for treating disease. The Egyptian Ebers Papyrus, discovered in a tomb near Luxor, listed many prescriptions made of hundreds of substances from plants, animals, and minerals.

Hippocrates classified herbs into hot and cold and moist and dry, and listed 300-400 species of effective medicinal plants. Aristotle compiled a list of medicinal plants, and his student Theophrastus explained their effects on humans and animals and established the science of botany with his descriptions of medicinal plants growing in Athens.

Dioscorides, the Roman army physician, wrote *De Materia Medica* (60 CE), a five-volume work in Greek, compiling approximately 500 plants and preparations of about 1000 drugs. Abdullah Al Bitar (1021–1080 CE), an Arabic botanist and pharmaceutical scientist, wrote the *Explanation of Dioscorides Book on Herbs*, and later, *The Glossary of Drugs and Food Vocabulary*, which contained the names of 1400 drugs. Although awareness of medicinal benefits of mint dates to the first century CE, in Elizabethan times, more than 40 ailments were reported to be remedied by mint, which is still used today in home therapies and in pharmaceutical preparations to relieve stomach and intestinal cramps.

The Coca plant is indigenous to South America and its leaves have been used in folk medicine in the Andes for thousands of years, both as a general stimulant and for medical purposes. Chewing the sacred coca leaf induced a mild, long-lasting euphoria. The Incas revered coca and used it in magical ceremonies and initiation rites. The plant has played an important part in modern society. Local anesthetics such as lidocaine are cocaine derivatives. The original recipe for Coca-Cola, that was invented in 1885 by John Pemberton, contained cocaine.

Another powerful natural drug originates from the humble poppy. Heroin, morphine, and other opiates trace their origins to this plant. The earliest cultivation of opium poppies was in Mesopotamia, around 3400 BCE. Opium use in ancient Egypt flourished during the reign of King Tutankhamen. Other civilizations used opium to induce sleep and relieve pain. In 1803, morphine was one of the earliest drugs to be isolated from the opium plant. Today, opiates—both synthetic and natural—hold great sway in modern society, though their prescription has become controversial.

Leaves and bark of willow trees, found in moist soils of cold temperate regions, have been mentioned in ancient texts from Mesopotamia to Egypt. Hippocrates wrote extensively about their medicinal properties. The Ebers Papyrus mentioned certain species of willow for three specific remedies. Willow bark is an herbal preparation that is available today in tablets over the counter. It is better known in a different form, however: In 1852, Salicin was synthesized from willow bark. The drug company Bayer modified it into acetylsalicylic acid (Aspirin), which reduces fever, inflammation, and pain. It is one of the most widely used medications globally, with an estimated 44,000 tons and 50-120 billion pills consumed annually, often to prevent arterial blood clotting. In fact, approximately 40 percent of all medications sold at pharmacies today are derived from plants, including the 20 most popular prescription drugs in the US.

Heart failure therapies were revolutionized by William Withering's discovery of the therapeutic properties of the Digitalis purpurea flower, which brought about a medical breakthrough saving countless lives. Withering, an English physician and botanist, tested the purple foxglove flower *Digitalis purpurea* and recognized the active ingredient, now known as digoxin, has a therapeutic effect on patients with dropsy or accumulation of fluid in legs caused by congestive heart failure. Though toxic in high doses, in milder doses, heart muscle contractions increase, and the body rids itself of excess fluid, while regulating heartbeats.

The phrase "patent medicine" emerged in the late 17th century for the marketing of medical elixirs. Those favored with royalties were issued statements authorizing their use and advertising. Few, if any nostrums were patented. Chemical patents would begin to be issued in the US in 1925, requiring disclosure of ingredients, which most promoters of elixirs avoided.

In the 1800s, patent medicine became more commonly used in the US for pills and tonics to cure and prevent all diseases from headaches to cancer and infections from venereal diseases to tuberculosis. Some helped with pain relief and contained alcohol or cocaine, while others functioned purely as placebos. The advertising industry marketed these using implausible claims that they were panaceas. Another publicity stunt for promoting these drugs was the "medicine show", a traveling circus that employed a "muscle man" as a stooge who touted the cure-all medicines as the source of his powers. Later, a few radioactive medicines containing uranium or radium were also marketed. Journalists began informing the public about the danger of using these drugs and the potential for addiction or death. Morris Fishbein, a physician, and editor of the Journal of the American Medical Association, in the first half of the 20th century, dedicated much of his career to exposing pseudoscientific practices and driving quacks out of business.

Morris was not alone in seeking to uncover such charlatans. Samuel Adams was an American investigative journalist who, in 1905, was hired by *Collier's* magazine to write series of articles about patent medicine. He published a well-read article under the title "The Great American Fraud" that exposed false claims made about patent medicines, pointing out that some of them were actually harmful to one's health. The series had a huge impact, ultimately leading to the passage of the Pure Food and Drug Act of 1906. To this day, the regulation and investigation of medicines is a crucial means of harm avoidance. In his book *Do You Believe in Magic? The Sense and Nonsense of Alternative Medicine* (2013), Paul Offit affirmed that vitamins and dietary supplements are far from panacea; in high doses, they have serious side effects that are harmful.

Alternative Medicine

Unlike complimentary treatment, which is used alongside conventional medicine, alternative medicine is employed as a substitute for orthodox medical practice. Examples of complimentary treatments are biofeedback, hypnosis, meditation, and yoga; meanwhile, examples of alternative medicine are homeopathy, which will be discussed later, and chiropractic. Patients are driven to these latter remedies to avoid surgery or visit physicians. Many researchers believe that the primary benefit of these remedies is the placebo effect. Morris Fishbein was vilified by the chiropractic community for his campaigning to suppress and end chiropractic as a profession and label it as a pseudoscience.

Chiropractic began in the US in 1895 with the Canadian-American **Daniel (DD) Palmer**, a former beekeeper, who claimed to have improved a man's hearing by manipulating his back. Palmer stated that he first received the idea of chiropractic from the spirit of a diseased physician. He believed that the cause of every disease, including smallpox, is the subluxation of the spinal column. Today, chiropractic is widely considered a healthcare discipline that treats musculoskeletal pain and other conditions with manipulation of the spine and other joints. Americans love chiropractors, and more than 35 million people in the US visit a chiropractor annually with over two-thirds seeking support for lower back pain. There are over 70,000 chiropractors currently registered in the US who perform one million chiropractic adjustments every day. Many patients report favorable responses to these manipulations. A number of fatal and severe complications, though rare, have been reported in scientific journals after manipulating the cervical spine. Debate continued today about the degree of placebo effect in chiropractic treatment, nevertheless.

Epidemics

Throughout history epidemics of diseases and pandemics, crossing international boundaries, plagued humanity killing millions of people. Bacteria or viruses can elicit these calamities. Caused by more than one organism including smallpox and typhus, the plague of Athens (430 BCE) was the earliest recorded pandemic infecting most of the population killing one quarter of its people. Later the Antonine Plaque may have contributed to the decline and fall of the Roman Empire. Six of the most consequential disease outbreaks and their impact will be chronicled.

Bubonic Plague (1347-50) was the largest of three similar pandemics and nick-named the 'Black Death.' It killed over 50 million people—a whole third of Europe's population—making it the worse pandemic in human history. This is largely because antibiotic treatment was not available at the time. The disease came to the US during the third wave of the pandemic in 1900 and was brought by rats on ships, affecting the rural west and southwestern states. Its origin, the *Yersinia pestis* bacteria, was discovered in the late 19th century to be carried through rodents and fleas. Infected people developed swellings (buboes) in lymph nodes of armpits and groins and sometimes the black tissue gangrene which gave it its name; without treatment, many die from septicemia or pneumonia. Transmission may also occur by handling tissue or blood from an infected animal or inhalation of infected droplets. Sadly, countries have used the plague as a biological weapon, intentionally triggering epidemics.

Malaria is an ancient disease mentioned even in Mesopotamian clay tablets and found in ancient Egyptian mummies. Disease outbreaks continued to be reported for the following 2000 years, and historians speculate that repeated Malaria epidemics affected ancient Greece In Europe, malaria flourished in crowded settlements where there was standing water during the warm seasons. Malaria was imported to the New World by African slaves who were immune to the disease, thanks to longstanding genetic defenses and lifelong exposure. The disease weakened Civil War soldiers and infected presidents from Washington to Lincoln. Without access to modern insect repellents, German troops during World War I in East Africa suffered heavy casualties from malaria. According to the WHO, in 2019, more than 229 million people are still contracting malaria, leading to approximately 409,000 deaths worldwide; over 95% of these deaths occurred in

Africa, where the disease is endemic. Malaria symptoms include fever, vomiting, and headaches, and in severe cases, jaundice, seizures, coma, or death ensue. Charles Laveran, a French army doctor, first identified the disease's crescent-shaped bodies in 1880 while in Algeria looking through a crude microscope at blood cells from a febrile soldier. In 1897, British surgeon Ronald Ross discovered that malaria parasites grew in mosquitos. Malaria is, in fact, caused by single-celled microorganisms, the *Plasmodium* group, and triggered by infected female mosquito bites, which introduce the organisms to the blood and liver. In 1820, the French chemists Joseph Pelletier and Jean Caventou isolated quinine from cinchona tree bark, which became a therapy used worldwide. In 1934, the synthesis of chloroquine as an antimalarial drug marked a milestone in controlling epidemics. Of all drugs manufactured to date, chloroquine and artemisinin are the two most popularly used today. Recently, a promising vaccine has also been developed for disease prevention for vulnerable African children.

Cholera is a small intestine infection from the bacterium *Vibrio cholera*, which produces toxins. Within hours of exposure, it induces watery diarrhea, vomiting, and muscle cramps—along with severe dehydration and electrolyte imbalance. The word 'cholera' came from Greek, meaning "bile," but the disease originated on the Indian subcontinent and continues to be prevalent in that region. The disease was referenced in European literature as early as 1642, by the Dutch physician Jakob de-Bondt. In 1854, a cholera epidemic struck England leading British physician John Snow to argue the disease was not airborn but sprang from bodies of water, especially cesspools. In the same year, Italian physician and anatomist Filippo Pacini discovered the organism, which caused the disease: *Vibrio cholera*.

The cholera bacteria itself is found in shellfish but also transmitted through contaminated food or water. Houseflies are suspected of transmitting at least 65 diseases to humans, including: anthrax, cholera, dysentery, leprosy, typhoid fever, yaws, tularemia, and tuberculosis.

The most recent cholera pandemic in the United States started in 1961. Cholera still exists, however, in Africa, Southeast Asia, and Haiti. Several antibiotics are effective against cholera. With timely treatment most patients will survive, but without treatment, mortality rates are around 50%. The Spanish physician Jaume Ferran developed a cholera inoculation in 1885, which was the first to immunize humans against a bacterial disease. Cholera vaccines are given by mouth and provide protection for about six months.

Typhoid fever, caused by *Salmonella typhi* bacteria, is a serious health threat, especially dangerous among children. It is contagious but can also come from contaminated food and water. Symptoms develop slowly—sometimes weeks after exposure. They include high fever, headache, stomach pain, constipation, diarrhea, and skin rashes. The disease triggers a high fever and gastrointestinal symptoms that may cause bowel perforation and death. French doctors Pierre Bretonneau and Pierre Louis described typhoid fever as a specific disease, unique from typhus. The disease has continued to affect populations in the 20th Century, with 54 outbreaks since 1950. One of the biggest typhoid fever epidemics occurred between 1906 and 1907 in New York. Antibiotic treatment is effective, and vaccines are partially effective—though usually reserved for travelers to areas where the disease is prevalent.

Mary Mallon (1869–1938), or Typhoid Mary, was an Irish-born American cook who infected dozens of people with typhoid fever while working for families, causing three confirmed deaths. She was the first person identified in the US to be an asymptomatic carrier of typhoid bacteria **(Fig 6)**. She persisted working as a cook, thereby exposing others to the disease. Because of her insistence to continue working she was forcibly quarantined twice by authorities. Eventually, for the final two decades of her life she was confined to North Brother Island. Mallon died after a total of nearly 30 years in isolation. Her nickname

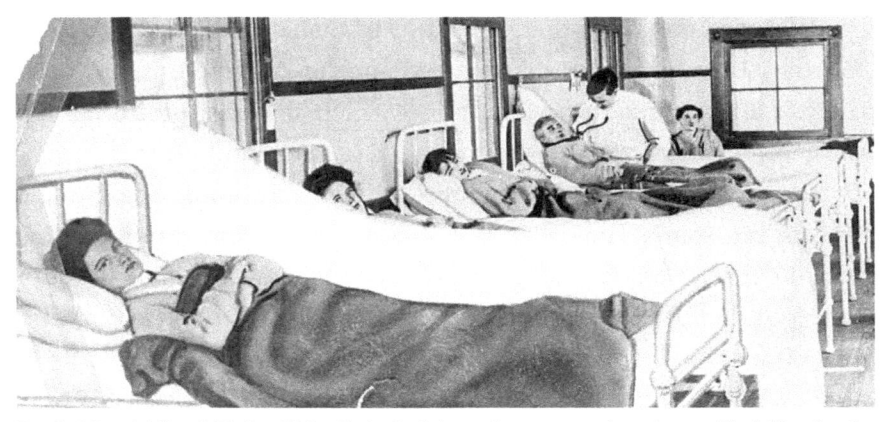

Fig 6. Mary Mallon "Typhoid Mary", the Irish-born American cook, in hospital bed (front), who was the first known asymptomatic carrier of the disease infecting dozens of people. (Wikipedia)

has since gained currency as a term for persons who spread misfortune, unaware that they are doing so.

Yellow fever is an infectious viral disease transmitted by a female mosquito bite. The infection can be mild or severe and potentially fatal. It causes internal bleeding and kidney and liver damage that results in jaundice—or yellow discoloration of skin and eye—giving it its name. In most cases, symptoms include fever, chills, loss of appetite, nausea, muscle pains, and headaches. The disease originated in central Africa and was initially brought to the New World by the slave trade. In the US, there were thirty-five yellow fever epidemics between 1702 and 1800, and from 1800 to 1879, there was nearly an epidemic every year. The 1793 Philadelphia yellow fever epidemic caused mass exodus of 20,000 people from the city. In 2013, yellow fever infected about 127,050 and caused 45,000 deaths worldwide, with nearly 90 percent of these in Africa. There is no specific treatment for yellow fever other than alleviating the symptoms with rest, fluids and cough medicine. Yellow fever virus was the first human virus to be isolated in 1927. Vaccination programs for yellow fever are used worldwide as effective disease prevention measures.

Poliomyelitis is another viral disease that causes crippling muscle paralysis; it has affected humanity since prehistoric times. Muscle paralysis affects limbs or whole body, which impedes breathing and whose only treatment was an iron lung, a machine invented, in the 1940s and 50s, by Americans Philip Drinker and Louis Shaw to aid patients' breathing. The device was necessary for a few months during the acute disease phase, and most patients were weaned; some lived for the rest of their lives in an iron lung, and one patient reported to be in it for 60 years. Poliomyelitis is now nearly extinct.

As we will see in later chapters, several immigrant physicians were instrumental in discovering the cause of some of these epidemics and developing therapies for their control and cure.

Medical Breakthroughs

Five momentous medical breakthroughs took place in the 19th century and changed medicine forever, namely: x-ray, antiseptic, anesthesia, antibiotics, and vaccines.

X-Ray

German physicist Wilhelm Roentgen discovered X-rays using glass tubes in 1895. He first took an image of his wife Emma's hand. For his discovery, he won the first Nobel Prize for Physics. French physicist Henry Becquerel discovered radioactivity in 1896 in uranium which emits radiation—like X-rays, but more powerful. Becquerel was awarded half of the Nobel Prize for Physics in 1903, the other half being given to Pierre and Marie Curie for their study of the Becquerel radiation. The Curies discovered radium and found it one million times more radioactive than pure uranium and can destroy human tissue; radioactive material was later used to eradicate cancer cells. X-rays became quintessential to diagnosing many diseases and injuries.

Antiseptics

The story of antisepsis is the story of practicing hygiene, preventing infections and saving limbs and lives. It is a narrative of five European physicians.

During the Renaissance, the French barber surgeon Ambroise Pere (1510–1590) could not enter medical school because he did not know Latin. Therefore, he joined the 'Hotel Dieu' (Hotel-of-God) in Paris, one of the oldest known hospitals in the world that was for charity. There, he sharpened his surgical skills and became one of the most influential doctors of his time. As a military surgeon he abandoned the practice of pouring boiling oil on battle wounds, instead dressing the gunshot wounds with homemade ointment that proved less painful and more effective in minimizing infection than searing wounds. Also, instead of using a crude hot iron to stop bleeding from amputation stumps, he used thread to sew up bleeding vessels. Pere published *Method of Treating Wounds* (1545), thus pioneering this gentler method of handling tissues. His 26 French books were compiled into one volume (1575), which at first was not accepted by the medical community but later was translated to Latin.

In 1756, British physician Percival Pott (1714–1788) sustained an open fracture of his leg—a serious injury that often resulted in infection and death. Amputation was suggested to him, but he refused and splinted the leg, keeping the wound clean and preventing infection, ultimately allowing the fracture to heal. Later, his method of keeping wounds clean to prevent infection became accepted practice across the medical establishment. Pott introduced other methods, to prevent infection of burn wounds. In 1775, an outbreak of cancer of the scrotum occurred in Britain and was thought to have come from venereal disease. During that year, Pott noticed that cancer of the scrotum developed among many young chimney sweep boys and doubted the condition was sexually transmitted, but rather suggested it came from the chimney soot trapped in the scrotal skin—this was the earliest report on occupational disease. After Pott's publication, more cases emerged which influenced a change in public policy by initiating a series of "Chimney Sweepers' Acts," which aimed to protect young chimney sweepers and led to a decline in scrotal cancer. Pott died and did not live to see the influence of his work. His revelation raised awareness that certain cancers can be prevented by eliminating carcinogens; one example of this is the link between tobacco and lung cancer. More carcinogens were recognized later, including asbestos, Agent Orange pesticide, and ultraviolet rays.

Hygiene practices have been limited in medical establishments until the modern era. Until the 19th century, doctors did not wash their hands before surgery—a trend that contributed to frequent infections after operations. Puerperal fever, a deadly infection of the uterus, occurred after childbirth, and was very common in Vienna's maternity wards. In 1847, the Hungarian obstetrician Ignaz Semmelweis became the first to advance the idea of "hand hygiene" and hand washing in obstetric clinics to prevent the spread of infections. Implementing this practice substantially dropped the incidence of deadly puerperal fever. Semmelweis did not have an explanation for his observation, which conflicted with the medical opinions of the time; his ideas were consequently rejected by the medical community. He suffered a nervous breakdown and was committed to an asylum, where he was beaten by the guards and developed a gangrenous wound infection on his hand that ironically resulted in his death. Semmelweis became known as the "savior of mothers." William Halsted, the Johns Hopkins Hospital's first surgeon-in-chief, is credited as the first to develop and introduce rubber surgical gloves in the US in 1894 to be used by surgeons to prevent infection.

Robert Koch, a German country doctor, who supported the germ theory and was able to grow bacteria in culture medium, proving that bacteria are the cause of diseases like tuberculosis. He identified the anthrax bacteria, Bacillus anthracis, in the blood of sick livestock in the 1880s, which can infect people who come into contact with infected animals causing skin ulcers, shortness of breath, nausea and vomiting, and abscess formation. Despite causing hundreds of thousands of deaths annually until the 20th century, the disease is rare in the US today. Unfortunately, anthrax has been developed as a germ weapon by several countries. Antibiotics are effective in preventing and treating the disease. Pasteur's vaccine also played a role in preventing anthrax among livestock and humans.

Joseph Lister observed in 1865 that open wounds become infected but covered wounds do not, and he began to explore the potential of antibacterial chemicals in preventing wound infection. He used carbolic acid to treat open wounds and fractures, preventing infection and introducing the concept of antiseptic surgery. His idea was initially rejected by many surgeons, but after lecturing about his discovery during a visit to the US in 1886, his method was adopted in major centers such as Johns Hopkins Hospital. Lister ushered in the age of antisepsis and antiseptic surgery.

Anesthesia
Successful uses of anesthesia have remained limited until relatively in recent history. Using snow as anesthetic was attempted in 1807 by French army surgeon Dominique Larrey who noticed the pain from limb amputation was lessened by the application of snow. In 1812, during the battle of Borodino, Larrey performed more than 200 amputations within 24 hours, as well as a further 300 amputations in the battle of Berezina. He used snow to anesthetize amputation stumps. Later, other surgeons accepted the concept of cold anesthesia.

Humphry Davy, a British chemist, discovered nitrous oxide in 1799, and noticed that it made him laugh—hence the nickname he gave to it: "laughing gas." He wrote about its potential anesthetic properties and pain relief qualities for surgery. Nitrous oxide anesthesia continues to be used today in surgery.

At Massachusetts General Hospital, on October 16th, 1846, a group of physicians gathered in an operating amphitheater and Boston dentist William Morton placed an inhaler with ether on a patient's face while a surgeon proceeded to remove a tumor from the patient's neck. The patient was asleep and, when awakened was not aware that he had surgery; this ushered in the modern age of anesthesia and truly painless surgery. Prior to that momentous day, Morton used ether on his dog, which did not respond to a pinprick while asleep. Next, he tried it on himself and—after taking a deep breath of ether—he woke up a whole 8 minutes later. Charles Jackson also claimed that he was the first to use ether; he and Morton quarreled over the issue. However, Crawford Long from Georgia was, in fact, the very first to use it in 1842, though he did not publicize it. The Massachusetts General Hospital committee studied the matter and ruled that Morton (not Jackson) should be credited for the invention of painless surgery. Morton would, in fact, later die of a stroke following a fit of anger on reading a newspaper article crediting Jackson. Jackson himself would later go insane and was found at a cemetery after reading Morton's tombstone: *William C G Morton Inventor of anesthetic inhalation.* Jackson was taken to a lunatic asylum where he would eventually die; controversy and conflict killed both men.

James Simpson was a Scottish obstetrician who did not approve of ether as anesthetic because of its odor and combustibility. In 1847, he discovered chloroform—which was a sweet-smelling noncombustible liquid. Chloroform was used for some time but later found to have adverse effects and was not the most effective anesthetic. Similarly, in the 1950s, nonflammable halothane anesthetic was discovered in Britain and became popular, but it was later abandoned because of its side effects.

Antibiotics and vaccines

Infections have plagued humanity since the beginning of our very existence, their cause and cure proving ever elusive. Infections often led to fatal epidemics worldwide. Attempts to curb infectious spreads were unsuccessful initially—until vaccinations and antibiotics were invented.

The arrival of Europeans in the New World brought new infectious diseases that decimated the population of the Natives; among those is the smallpox. English Lady Mary Montagu the wife of the British Ambassador to the Ottoman Empire witnessed, in 1717, while living there, the locals using of smallpox vaccination. Upon her return to England she introduced and advocated for smallpox vaccination.

In the late 1700s, smallpox epidemics swept through Europe and proved even deadlier than cholera, bubonic plague, or yellow fever. If the patient survived, he would have vision or hearing impairments and horrific skin scars but will develop permanent immunity against the disease. In 1796, British physician Edward Jenner created the world's first successful smallpox vaccine. He noticed that people infected with cowpox were immune to smallpox. He expanded on this observation by inoculating 8-year-old James Phipps with fluid collected from a cowpox sore on the hand of a milkmaid, rendering him immune to the virus, despite a brief, mild illness. Thousands of people were vaccinated, including the British Royal family and Napoleon's soldiers. In the colonial United States, inoculation became a political issue with those advocating for and against vaccination, especially for yellow fever. However, after losing a battle over British-occupied Canada, partly because of a smallpox outbreak in camps, George Washington had his soldiers inoculated. Natives in the United States who were inoculated benefited from Jenner's invention, which lessened the impact of the "white man's disease" which had previously decimated native populations.

It would be another hundred years before the full potential of vaccination was discovered, however. In 1885, after intensive research,

Louis Pasteur injected the first of 14 doses of rabbit spinal cord fluid containing inactivated rabies virus into 9-year-old Joseph Meister, who had been bitten by a rabid dog, two days earlier. The otherwise inevitable death of the boy was prevented; the rabies vaccine ushered in a new modern era of immunization. Pasteur also developed a vaccine against cholera. In 1884, Spanish physician Jaume Ferran developed a live vaccine isolated from cholera patients that he used on more than 30,000 patients during that year's epidemic. Later, based on Pasteur 's work, the anthrax vaccine for humans was developed in Britain and Russia. A polio vaccine for humans was later developed in the 20th century.

Further pharmaceutical drugs would be developed in the Twentieth Century. Paul Ehrlich, a German physician in 1909, discovered that a chemical called arsphenamine was an effective treatment for syphilis. Ehrlich referred to his discovery as "chemotherapy." Alexander Fleming, a Scottish physician later accidently discovered penicillin in 1928. He noticed that a fungus, *Penicillium notatum*, had contaminated a culture plate of *Staphylococcus* bacteria he had left uncovered. The fungus created a bacteria-free zone wherever it grew on the plate. Fleming isolated the mold in a pure culture that is effective in preventing *Staphylococcus* growth even when diluted 800 times, with no toxic effect. During the 'D-Day' landings in 1944, where British and American troops began to expel the Nazis from Northern France, penicillin was widely used to treat troops for infections. By the end of World War II, penicillin was nicknamed a "wonder drug" for saving so many lives. Howard Florey and Ernst Chain, two scientists in Oxford, shared the 1945 Nobel Prize in Medicine with Alexander Fleming for their role in creating the first ever mass-produced antibiotic. German physician Gerhard Domagk also discovered a sulfa drug in 1935 that also became a popular antibiotic. For his discovery, he was awarded the 1939 Nobel Prize in Physiology or Medicine.

The Ukrainian-American inventor, biochemist, and microbiologist **Selman Waksman** (1888–1973), who discovered over 20 antibiotics, was the first to coin the term "antibiotic." Waksman was born in Nova Pryluka, Kiev—then part of the Russian Empire, now Ukraine—and emigrated to the US in 1910. He studied bacteriology and obtained a master's degree from Rutledge University and was later appointed as a research fellow at the University of California, Berkeley, receiving a Doctorate in Philosophy in Biochemistry. Waksman's team discovered several antibiotics, including actinomycin and neomycin. Although Waksman worked on streptomycin, which was effective against tuberculosis, Albert Schatz claimed to be the inventor of the medicine. Eventually, both Schatz and Waksman agreed to receive joint recognition as inventors of streptomycin. In 1952, however, Waksman was announced as the sole winner of the Nobel Prize in Physiology or Medicine for his discovery of streptomycin.

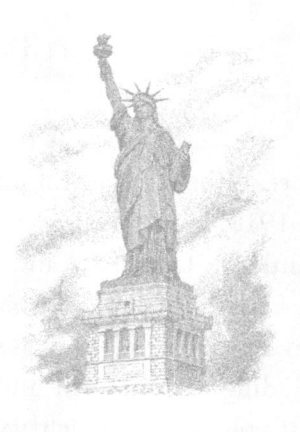

CHAPTER 2

Anatomical Science and Anatomists

Anatomy is the branch of medical science that deals with the study of the structure and organization of living organisms. It is concerned with the identification and description of the various parts of the body, including organs, tissues, and systems, and their relationships with each other. The study of anatomy is essential to understanding of physiology, which is the study of how these structures and systems function in a living organism. Anatomical knowledge is also important in the diagnosis and treatment of various medical conditions, as well as in the development of new medical technologies and procedures.

Anatomy is the heart of medicine; earlier medical advancements were only possible when anatomical knowledge became accessible. Many physicians' anatomists especially those in the Medieval Islamic era and later in Europe dared to break the taboos of their time and dissect the human body and make boundless anatomical discoveries. European and American physicians struggled to professionalize the practice of anatomy and christened it science to be incorporated in medical educational curricula.

Ancient Anatomists

Ancient Egyptian priests were the earliest known anatomists who acquired knowledge of human internal organs while embalming mummies. There was no paucity of physicians and students of anatomy in Ancient Greece, as we have discussed earlier, most of whom gravitated to the great medical school of Alexandria for their training. In Alexandria, around 280 BCE, two Greek physician-anatomists, Herophilus (335–280 BCE) and Erasistratus (304–250 BCE), were the earliest to perform human body dissections in a systematic manner. Herophilus challenged the authorities by becoming the first to perform public dissections of cadavers, where he described the function of the eye, heart, liver, pancreas, prostate, sex organs, salivary glands, and genital organs. He described and named the duodenum, part of the intestine at the lower end of the stomach. Herophilus deserves the honor of being recognized as the seminal father of anatomy. Erasistratus made similar anatomical descriptions and added important information about heart valves, skeletal muscles, nerves and their roles in motor and sensory control through the brain. He is credited as the first to describe the cerebrum and cerebellum components of the brain in some depth. Together, these physicians established the school of anatomy in Alexandria, which enhanced the growth of medical sciences.

Claudius Galen (129 CE–216 CE), of Pergamon, the Greek surgeon, was born in Turkey, studied medicine in Alexandria, and traveled extensively before settling in Rome. Human dissection was illegal in Rome at the time so Galen's anatomical research was based on dissecting dogs, pigs, and monkeys. During the Roman Empire, 130 CE, he performed live dissections on animals and was the first to demonstrate that nerves control muscles and that the larynx generates voice. He tied up the ureter and noticed that the kidney became enlarged and urine flow ceased. Galen then began to learn of human anatomy by peering into the bodies of injured gladiators. His anatomical knowledge helped him become one of the greatest surgeons of his time.

Galen wrote medical treatises based on animal dissection and applied the results to humans. He detailed the anatomy of the trachea—the windpipe. His contributions to the circulatory system differentiated venous (dark) and arterial (bright) blood. He argues that the blood passes through the cardiac ventricular septum—which remained unchallenged until Ibn al-Nafis, the Arabic physician, first described the process of pulmonary circulation.

From his anatomical knowledge, Galen also learned a great deal of physiology and was able to decipher a difficult case and make one of his most famous discoveries. Eudemus, the Roman physician, had developed a weakness and numbness in his ring and small fingers, and no one knew the cause. Galen attributed the symptoms to a prior neck injury and nerve damage. Galen's fame spread, and the emperor Marcus Aurelius retained him as his personal physician. Galen was also a philosopher and wrote a treatise entitled *That the Best Physician Is Also a Philosopher*. Galen's ideas, philosophy, and writings continued to monopolize key texts for physicians throughout the Arabic world and Middle Ages.

During the Medieval Islamic era, several other physicians also left their marks on the science of anatomy. Most Arabic and Persian medical encyclopedias had sections on anatomy with detailed schematic diagrams. Some of these practitioners were mentioned earlier—including Avicenna, al-Razi, and Ibn al-Nafis, who was the first to describe the anatomy of pulmonary circulation. Besides studying the composition of the whole body, eye anatomy, function and surgery were areas of interest to several Islamic physicians, some of whom wrote textbooks with descriptions of varied ophthalmic procedures.

Very little is known of Ammar ibn Ali al Mawsili, other than he was born in Mosul, Iraq, and traveled to Palestine and Egypt, where he gained knowledge of eye anatomy and practiced medicine and ophthalmology. He wrote "The book of choice in ophthalmology", became a renowned Arab oculist and is credited with inventing the hypodermic syringe, for the purpose of removing cataracts, a major cause of blindness.

Kamal Ali ibn Isa al Kahhal (940-1010 CE) was one of the most celebrated Arab ophthalmologists and was known as "the oculist". He authored the "Memorandum of Oculists", the most comprehensive and influential Arabic ophthalmology text to survive from the medieval era. The book details the eye's anatomy with illustrations of many diseases and remedies—with and without surgery. Among several conditions he described was 'uveitis' or inflammation of the eye, as well as 'epiphora' or excessive tearing (crocodile tears) of the eye. He noticed that epiphora resulted from overzealous cautery of an eye growth causing obstruction of tear ducts and suggested surgical treatment for the condition.

Hasan ibn al-Haytham, (al-Hazen), (965 CE-1040 CE) was an Iraqi physician who lived most of his life in Cairo, he explained that the eye is an optical instrument and meticulously described eye's anatomy. He developed theories about visual perception suggesting that images are formed when light is reflected by an object, passes through the eye, and relayed to the brain. In his "Book of Optics", he accurately drew the human eye with its optic nerves, chiasm, and bifurcation reaching the brain. For his seminal descriptions of eye anatomy and function, Al-Haytham is often referred to as "the father of modern optics."

Abd al-Latif al-Baghdadi (1162–1231), made dissections of many human skeletons during a famine in Egypt. He described the bones of the lower jaw and sacrum and corrected some of Galen's teaching. His reputation extended throughout Europe. His Arabic manuscript was discovered in 1665 and was translated into Latin in 1800.

Mansur ibn Ilyas, was a late 14th century and early 15th century Persian physician, known for publishing the first colored atlas of the human body. Its title translates as "The Anatomy of the Human Body", but it is known as "Mansur's Anatomy." It illustrates full pages of skeleton, muscles, nerves, vessels, and internal organs. He is also credited with one of the earliest anatomical sketches of a pregnant woman.

Dissection of human cadavers—a hallmark of the Alexandrian school of anatomy— declined after 200 CE because of religious prohibitions. When these bans were temporarily lifted, the Italian Mondino de Luzzi, restored anatomy and performed his first public dissection in Bologna in 1315 to medical students and spectators. He offered practical classes in his residence and wrote a new manual for anatomical dissection.

There are two other Italians, however, whose artistic genius is linked to anatomical knowledge. Leonardo DaVinci was not a physician, but in the 1490s, he secretly studied anatomy and made anatomical drawings of the human body. He spent late night hours hurrying through dissections before decay set into the corpses. He began creating a treatise on human anatomy with an extensive set of drawings—but the work was never published. He made the very first drawing of a late trimester fetus and of limbs with their muscles, nerves, and vessels. In the Vitruvian Man, DaVinci used the principles of geometry to explore the configuration of the human body. Through his art, da Vinci fostered scientific attitudes towards the study of anatomy. Equally, artist Michelangelo Buonarotti, Da Vinci's contemporary, also studied human form and performed anatomical dissections. He studied surface anatomy and drew illustrations from human models that reflected his detailed knowledge of the human structure.

Italian anatomist Bartolomeo Eustachio (1510?–1574) helped by painter Pietro da Cortona made masterful anatomical sketches of the human body, creating 47 engravings that render muscles, brain, spinal cord, and other internal organs. Eustachio described a duct that connects the nasopharynx to the middle ear that now carries his name. Another Italian, Hieronymus Fabricius (1533–1619), studied medicine in Padua, the site of a renowned medical center, and became a pioneer teacher, anatomist, and surgeon. In 1594, Fabricius revolutionized anatomical teaching when he designed the first theater for public anatomy dissections. He made exhaustive anatomical descriptions of the brain and became known as father of embryology.

Anatomist and physician Andreas Vesalius (1514 – 1564) of Brussels went to Paris to study anatomy at the Hotel Dieu but was disenchanted with the conditions of the anatomy theater and its decaying cadavers. He stole a body of a hanged criminal and studied its skeleton. He earned a medical degree from Padua and decided to create his own anatomical charts and plates from dissected specimens. In 1543, he released his *De Humani Corporis Fabrica*, a book that marked the beginning of modern anatomical science. It was the first medical text, which is based on topographical anatomy and is one of the most celebrated texts in the history of medicine. The book contained 300 vibrant illustrations with a blend of exquisite art and science and accurate depictions of human anatomy in exhaustive detail, including the innermost structures of the nervous, vascular, muscular, and skeletal systems.

Vesalius used anatomical dissections as a primary teaching tool and debunked many beliefs of prior scholars, including Aristotle and Galen, as erroneous. He showed that blood does not pass through the heart's invisible pores. He identified the liver as having two lobes one on either side. Vesalius' challenge to Galen earned him many enemies, even though Galen's dissections had only been based on animals. Vesalius spent his remaining years distressed, defending his book against critics. He met a friend in Jericho on his way to the Holy Land of Jerusalem. No information remains as to where he died. Vesalius made a turning point in the accurate study of human anatomy and became known as the "founder of modern anatomy."

The Englishman William Harvey (1578 –1657) traveled to Padua to study medicine where Galileo was lecturing about the importance of experimentation for learning. Harvey was influenced by Galileo's method and went on to read Hippocrates, Galen, and Vesalius. Back in England, he conducted experiments and gained knowledge of the heart, circulation, and vascular system from anatomical dissections. He proved Galen wrong and introduced the notion of circulation—that blood moves in perpetual motion in a circle caused by the beating heart. Harvey wrote a book, *On the Motion of the Heart and Blood in Animals* (1628). His reputation grew, and he was assigned physician to the English King Charles I and James I. Anatomists created a growing demand for cadavers, which quickly outpaced supply. So, Harvey joined other surgeons of his time in seeking out grave robbers to help steal the corpses of recently deceased people. Harvey's love for anatomy compelled him to suppress his emotions and even participate in the gruesome dissections of his father's and sister's bodies.

Johann Wirsung (1589–1643) was a German anatomist who was a well-known dissector in Padua. He is famous for the discovery of the pancreatic duct in 1642, which became known as the "duct of Wirsung." He noticed the duct while dissecting a recently hanged man. The duct within the pancreas is connected to the bile duct, and both help drain their contents into the small intestine. In 1643, Wirsung was shot and murdered, and conflicting stories circulated about the murderer and the motive. One account suggested that his student Moritz Hoffmann was his killer because he claimed to have discovered the duct in a turkey a year before Wirsung.

William Cheselden, the English surgeon and teacher of anatomy, published his book *Osteographia or the Anatomy of Bones* (1733) and offered the first full description of the human and animals skeletal systems. His accurate scientific description of human bone structures is sometimes combined with dynamic postures such as praying, holding other bones, or leaning against large animal skulls. He was also a skillful eye surgeon credited with performing the first-known eye surgery in 1728, helping a boy with cataracts recover from blindness endured since birth.

Shortly after the publication of Cheselden's book, another physician made an even greater contribution to the science of anatomy through his drawings. Bernhard Albinus (1697-770) was a German-born Dutch prodigy who attended medical school at the age of twelve in the Netherlands and became a professor of anatomy at just age 24. Between 1719 and 1767, he authored several publications with illustrations of various systems of the human anatomy. He is best known for his *Tabulae sceleti et musculorum corporis humani*, an exquisitely illustrated volume that was first published in Leiden in 1747, a project that was time-consuming and required much money, labor, science, and artistry. Albinus collaborated on his project with an artist, Jan Wandelaar; the resulting tables depicted skeletons in lifelike poses with landscape backgrounds.

Anna Manzolini was one of the earliest known female anatomists, an intellect and the skilled collaborator of her husband Giovani, a professor of anatomy at the University of Bologna, Italy. After her husband's passing in 1755, she received a post at the University of Bologna as an anatomical demonstrator with access to cadavers from the Bologna Hospital. She became an internationally renowned anatomist, anatomical wax modeler, and anatomy lecturer at Bologna University.

The Scottish surgeon William Hunter trained in anatomy at St George's Hospital, London, and became a leading anatomy teacher. He was an exceptional obstetrician of his time. In 1748, he established William's anatomy school in Central London; and in 1768, he built the renowned anatomy theatre and museum where many famous British anatomists and surgeons of the day were trained. In 1774, he published his great work *Anatomia uteri umani gravidi* (The anatomy of the human gravid uterus). This work was conceived when he acquired a pregnant female corpse and studied it at a time when the fetus was considered a small adult. The plates were engraved by a medical artist and showed the precise anatomy of the pregnant woman and her fetus in the process of development. Hunter would become the physician to Queen Charlotte, wife of King George III. He wrote, "*Anatomy is the only solid foundation of medicine; it is to the physician and surgeon what geometry is to the astronomer. It discovers and ascertains truth, overturns superstition and vulgar error.*" William also helped train his renowned younger brother, John Hunter, as a brilliant surgeon.

John dissected more than 2000 cadavers over twelve winters. In 1764, John Hunter established his own anatomy school in London and built a collection of skeletons and other organs. He amassed 14,000 anatomical specimens of humans and other vertebrates. Today, the Hunterian Museum at the Royal College of Surgeons of England hosts John Hunter's anatomy and pathology collections. William Shipping of Philadelphia spent time with Hunter and returned to the US to give the first formal anatomy lecture, where he promoted the study of anatomy.

Astley Cooper (1768 – 1841) was a British physician who attended John Hunter's lectures and was a master anatomist before he became a surgeon. He was passionate about anatomy and regarded each day of his life as wasted if he went to bed at night without having dissected that day. To the delight of spectators, Cooper performed public dissections of executed criminals in London and gave public lectures on comparative anatomy. He became the organizer of a network of body snatchers and suppliers that sent him endless corpses and specimens. As a student, he became involved in body snatching himself, and later in his career, he supported the families of the gravediggers if they were jailed. Cooper campaigned for the legalization of dissection, which resulted in the passage of the 'Anatomy Act' in 1832.

Cooper's knowledge of vascular anatomy allowed him to be the first surgeon to tie the biggest artery, the abdominal aorta, and earned him the title "father of arterial surgery." Charles Huston developed a leaking iliac artery (a major branch of the aorta which supplies the leg). To save this man's life from fatal hemorrhage, Cooper ligated the aorta, stopped the bleeding, and the leg remained viable—because blood supply still reached the leg through other channels.

Struggle for the Soul of Anatomy

In the 1820s, a mania for anatomy was in full swing in Europe, and the same fever also caught on in the US. For religious and social reasons, anatomists and the public clashed over the legitimacy and proper place of anatomical knowledge and research in American society. Anatomists had the burden to prove their profession was worthy and morally acceptable. In the first two-thirds of the 19th century, three American anatomists—William Horner, Charles Knowlton, and Oliver Wendell Holmes, Sr—argued for the legitimacy of their discipline and the importance of anatomy to be professionalized and included in medical education requirements.

Anatomy eventually became an essential component of the medical education curriculum. American medical schools, by the 1850s, made anatomy courses a prerequisite for obtaining a medical degree. There were four medical schools in the US in 1800; this number increased to more than 160 by 1900. Between 1865 and 1890, the number of American medical schools doubled, and the need for cadavers increased. The supply did not meet the demand, and the paucity of bodies for teaching anatomy prospered the task of grave robbery. The practice of body snatching grew, and graves became a ready source for specimens. During the 18th and 19th centuries in the United Kingdom, 'resurrectionists' were body snatchers commonly employed by anatomists to exhume the bodies of the recently dead. The same practice was adopted in the US, where the luckiest medical schools sat adjacent to graveyards and churchyards. Black markets for bodies flourished and became a lucrative business. Grave robbers retrieved fresh bodies from coffins, placing them in whisky barrels to mask the smell, and shipped them in railroad to medical schools. People were even sometimes killed so their bodies could be sold. Boston and New York medical students became body snatchers, and in Baltimore, medical students adopted the practice even before Johns Hopkins medical school was opened in 1893. Burial grounds of the poor and marginalized such as African Americans were targeted.

Society did not view the corpse as a lifeless body but as an individual whose rights should be protected. Religious people perceived eviscerating the human body with a dissecting knife as non-Christian and against honoring the dead with a proper funerary and decent burial. The public was outraged and viewed anatomical dissection as butchery and the body should not be subject to scientific inquiry. Bodies of the rich were buried very deep and in lead-sealed coffins to deter grave robbers from stealing them. Graveyard vigils were held, and families guarded the graves of their recently deceased in shifts until the bodies decomposed and became useless for dissection.

Outraged citizens forced the government to enact legislation against grave robbers and body snatching. Anatomy riots even occurred against anatomists and physicians. At least twenty major mobs rose against American medical schools between 1765 and 1884. The most notable were the "resurrection riots" of 1788 in New York City, and New Haven in 1824. Storming medical schools and attacking physicians forced schools to close or relocate. Anatomists also lobbied, and anatomy acts were passed, allowing unclaimed bodies to be consigned to medical schools, sometimes paying outstanding taxes of the deceased to the government in exchange for their bodies. Massachusetts passed the Anatomy Act of 1831, which allowed dissection of unclaimed bodies of the homeless, insane, and imprisoned. Similar laws in most states allowed medical schools to appropriate bodies of homeless people for dissection. Some judges ordered criminals' bodies donated to medical schools after hanging. After all confrontations and legislations, the traffic of dead bodies finally ceased.

The Uniform Anatomical Gift Act of 1968 created the option to donate organs as a gift from a deceased person for surgical transplantation or saving lives. The same act in 2006, gave individuals a chance to make a voluntary gift of their bodies in case of an accident on the back of their driver's license; it also created donor registries. The American Association for Anatomy promoted body donation programs, which are now utilized in every medical and dental school as part of medical education. This association dictates that those entrusted with the responsibility of the program must meet the high standards of integrity, identity, and security for the bodies donated to their programs. It proposes guidelines for the ethical use of donated bodies, cadavers to be held in secured facilities without entry of unauthorized personnel and proper disposing of cadaveric remains.

Gray's anatomy textbook was first published in 1858 under the title *Anatomy: Descriptive and Surgical*. In 1938, it was abbreviated to *Gray's Anatomy*. Its 42nd edition was published in 2020. The British anatomists and surgeons Henry Gray and Henry Carter collaborated on publishing this text that achieved greater eminence and longevity than any other medical book in modern history. It remained today a standard reference to medical students and physicians. Gray's descriptions were exact, and Carter's drawings were exquisite. Gray contracted smallpox and died at age 34 before the publication of the second edition.

European and American artists immortalized anatomy. The anatomy lesson series were part of the Dutch Golden Age of Art. The first of these began with the work of Pieter Mierevelt who painted *Anatomy Lesson of Dr Willem van der Meer* (1617), which showed a doctor holding a knife over the open belly of a male cadaver with 15 people watching. The Dutch Rembrandt Van Rijn painted his masterpiece *Anatomy Lesson of Dr Tulp* (1632), which pictured the surgeon Nicolaes Tulp explaining the anatomy of the arm musculature to a group of doctors. Johannes Deijman was the subject of Rembrandt's second anatomy lesson, *Anatomical Lesson of Dr Deijman* (1656) which depicted the doctor dissecting the motionless brain of a hanged criminal. Dutch physician-anatomist Frederik Ruysch was the subject of two paintings of anatomy lessons: *The anatomy lesson of Professor Frederik Ruijsch* (1670), painted by Adriaen Backer showing Ruysch with dissecting instruments above an unopened corpse alongside six spectators; the second was by Johan van Neck (1683) and shows Ruysch dissecting the belly of a child with five onlookers. In the United States, Thomas Eakin painted the *Agnew Clinic* (1889) to honor anatomist and surgeon David Agnew who is depicted performing a mastectomy on a woman while medical students watch on attentively at Pennsylvania University.

Immigrant Anatomists

Most anatomists of the 18th and 19th centuries who made anatomical advances were Europeans from Italy, Germany, Britain, and France. A few were also United States immigrants who came mostly from Europe, becoming accomplished physician-anatomists and making key discoveries about the human internal organs. Five will be discussed: three from the British Isles, one Australian, and one from Austria.

In the second half of the 18th century, an Irish anatomist engaged in marketing his public anatomy lectures in New York by advertising them in newspapers, including the New York Gazette. His anatomical lectures and dissection of dead slaves—before the American Revolution—became very successful and earned him fame and fortune. His name is **Samuel Clossy** (1724-1786). He was born in Dublin, Ireland. After obtaining a Bachelor's Degree in Medicine and Surgery in 1751, he studied in London under the renowned anatomist William Hunter. He was then awarded a Medical Degree from Trinity College Dublin in 1755. While a practicing physician, he wrote *Observations on some of the diseases of the parts of the body; chiefly taken from the dissection of morbid bodies* (1763), considered one of the first systematic studies of pathology in the English language.

Clossy emigrated to New York in 1763 and lectured on anatomy, advertising his lectures. His successful lectures earned him employment as a tutor and professor of natural philosophy in 1765 at King's College (Columbia University). Two years later, he became the college's first professor of anatomy—and the first college professor in a medical subject in North America. Thus, he played a vital role in inaugurating New York's first medical school. During the Revolutionary War, he returned for a brief visit to England and Dublin, where he died. Few physicians during the colonial times brought such a wide knowledge of anatomy and disease as Clossy. His work in New York earned him a reputation as a pioneering anatomist. His published seminal observations on diseases were chiefly acquired from the dissection of "morbid bodies" and are considered one of the first systematic studies of pathology in the English language. Clossy was unanimously elected an honorary fellow of the Royal College of Physicians of Ireland.

While Clossy was dissecting the bodies of deceased patients to learn about the causes of death, he was in essence performing autopsies. Today, an autopsy is a medical procedure where a physician performs a detailed examination of a human corpse to determine the cause and time of death. All organs are removed, and each is inspected for signs of injury or disease by analyzing the contents of hollow organs.

In the early half of the 18th century, duels in the US were common. What was uncommon is for physicians to engage in them. An immigrant anatomist physician known for his temper participated in a duel in the US. Lucky for him, he survived the ordeal unscathed, whereas his opponent—ironically a seasoned brigadier general in the military—was wounded. This anatomist was **Granville Pattison** (1791–1851). Pattison grew up in Kelvingrove, Glasgow, and little is known about his childhood, though in adulthood he had a tendency to argue with colleagues. In 1813, Pattison was admitted to the Faculty of Physicians and Surgeons of Glasgow. He became an assistant lecturer of anatomy, physiology, and surgery at the Andersonian Institute—a position he resigned from a year later after a dispute with a colleague physician, Andrew Ure.

In 1818, Pattison immigrated to Philadelphia and lectured privately on anatomy, where he quarreled with physician Nathaniel Chapman—who later became founding president of the American Medical Association. In 1820, Pattison took the position of the chair of anatomy, physiology, and surgery at the University of Maryland, Baltimore but resigned after five years following a disagreement over his anatomical research and description of tissue in the male genitalia. This led him to fight in a duel with a military lawyer, General Thomas Cadwalader, whom he wounded with a pistol shot.

Pattison returned to England in 1827 and was appointed professor of anatomy at the University of London while acting as surgeon to the University Dispensary. He was coerced to relinquish his post under pressure from students and colleagues—who questioned his teaching methods. Pattison returned to Philadelphia, where he became professor of anatomy at Jefferson Medical College and received a Doctor of Medicine degree, later being appointed Professor of Anatomy at New York University, a post he retained till his death.

Pattison **(Fig 7)** was an accomplished academic writer. He authored *Experimental Observations on the Operation of Lithotomy* (1820), edited Allan Burns's *Observations on the Surgical Anatomy of the Head and Neck* (1823), the *American Recorder*, and the *Register and Library of Medical and Chirurgical Science*, among other publications. Pattison was a renowned anatomist and surgeon but will forever be remembered as the antagonist anatomist for his propensity for conflict on both sides of the Atlantic.

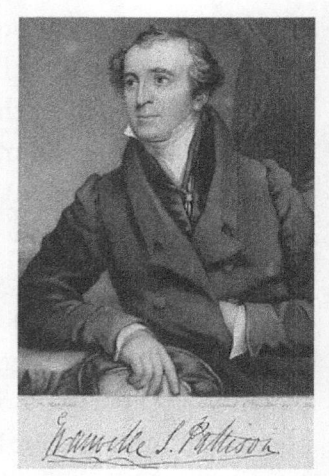

Fig 7. Scottish-American Granville Pattison, one of the earliest American academic anatomists, was chair of anatomy at the University of Maryland and later New York University. (Wikipedia)

Robley Dunglison (1798–1869) was a British-born physician and anatomist who came to the US upon a request from President Thomas Jefferson. The Board of the University of Virginia had commissioned Francis Gilmer to find professors in England for the new university. Gilmer offered Dunglison the anatomy and medicine professorship. In 1825, Dunglison arrived in Charlottesville, Virginia, to join the university faculty, where he became the first full-time professor of medicine in the US. Dunglison became a frequent visitor to Monticello, caring for Jefferson's health; and in 1826, was at the former president's deathbed.

Besides practicing medicine, Dunglison developed a strong interest in anatomy and made substantial contributions to human anatomy and physiology, both in Virginia and Maryland. He assembled a collection of materials for anatomical demonstrations and gave many courses in anatomy. A list of his anatomical dissections covered specimens from across the human body—including male and female reproductive systems, lungs, heart, brain, stomach, larynx, kidney, liver, and vascular system. Dunglison also focused on physiology, a subject related to anatomy, and took an active role in the scientific experiments on gastric digestion. When he requested a separate anatomical theater, Thomas Jefferson granted him the request and designed it in 1825. Dunglison published a landmark textbook *Human Physiology* (1832) that earned him the title "Father of American Physiology"; he was also an educator (Chapter 3).

The female reproductive organs remained something of a mystery to the medical community until the 19th century. The external female genitalia includes three main areas: the vaginal opening, clitoris, and labia—both outer (majora) and inner (minora). The vaginal tube is part of the internal genitalia, which also include the cervix, uterus, Fallopian tubes, and ovaries. Between the clitoris and the vaginal opening lies the urethral opening. The urethra is a tube, which is part of the urinary system; it excretes urine and extends from the bladder.

Two small glands located in the vaginal wall on either side of the female urethra have pinprick size openings. These pea-sized glands have mucous-based fluids which are ejaculated following sexual stimulation. This secretion is very important for lubricating the vagina during intercourse, but also acts as an antimicrobial to prevent urethral infections. An area behind these glands is surrounded by sensitive nerve endings, sometimes called the G spot and responsible for ejaculating a milky white fluid during orgasm.

The medical community and anatomists failed to recognize the presence of these two glands for many centuries; that is, until a Scottish physician and anatomist formally described them in 1880. This immigrant was **Alexander Skene** (1837–1900), who was born in Fyvie village in Aberdeenshire, Scotland. He attended King's College in London before arriving in Toronto, Canada, where he began studying medicine. Skene immigrated to the US in 1857 and continued his medical studies at the University of Michigan. He finally settled in Brooklyn, where he earned his medical degree in 1863 from the Long Island College Hospital (State University of New York). During the Civil War, Skene served as an assistant surgeon in the Union Army, stationed in South Carolina and New York. He helped create an army ambulance. After the war, he began teaching at Long Island College Hospital and eventually specialized in gynecology. He was appointed Professor of Women's Diseases at Long Island College Hospital in 1870, serving for nearly three decades.

Skene **(Fig 8)** was an educator, researcher, and prolific medical writer, authoring five textbooks and over 100 papers—many on anatomy. But his interest and study of anatomy led to his fame, particularly in the field of female pelvic anatomy, as he dissected the external genitalia resulting in a landmark article, *The anatomy and pathology of two important glands of the female urethra*, published in 1880. He emphasized these glands' pathology of inflammation and infection. This discovery earned them the name "Skene's glands." Infection of these glands is now termed 'skenitis' and can also develop into cancer. These glands are homologous to the prostate glands in males. Skene did not understand their function at the time, but their importance during sexual intercourse and the nature of their infection were later recognized.

In the late 1880s, Skene helped to found the American Gynecological Society, the first national organization in the world devoted to obstetrics and gynecology—serving as its president (1886–1887). Following Skene's death, his colleagues at Long Island College Hospital raised funds to erect a monument in his honor and commissioned an artist to construct the shrine. In 1905, a larger-than-life bronze bust was completed and sat atop a white marble obelisk in Grand Army Plaza.

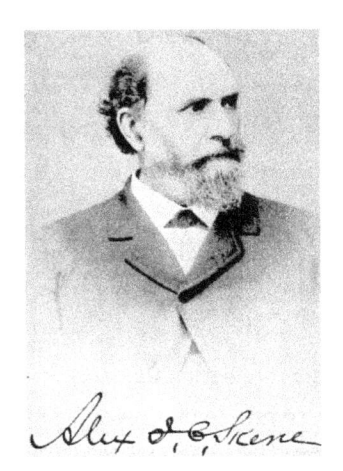

Fig 8. Scottish-American anatomist and gynecologist Alexander Skene who discovered the female genital glands that named after him. He founded the American Gynecological Society. (Wikipedia)

Nine years after Skene's passing, a boy was born in Perth, Australia. Although not a physician, he would later become an anatomist, histologist, primatologist, and nutritionist, producing pioneering work in anatomy that helped physicians understand the human physiology of the adrenal gland. His name was **Geoffrey Bourne** (1909–1988), and he would go on to receive a Doctor of Science degree from the University of Western Australia, alongside a Doctor of Philosophy award from Oxford University. He emigrated to the US and acquired citizenship in 1962. He became chairman of the anatomy department at Emory University in Atlanta. For sixteen years, he served as director of Yerkes Regional Primate Research Center and later became professor of nutrition at St. George's University School of Medicine, Grenada, West Indies.

Bourne's specialism would be the adrenal gland—a small triangular organ located above the kidney. This gland secretes hormones crucial to survival and daily bodily functions, including regulating metabolism and blood pressure in response to stress. While studying the anatomy of the mammalian adrenal gland, Bourne developed the first technique for demonstrating the presence of vitamin C in animal tissue in 1933. This made him a pioneer in the chemistry of cells and tissues and in the field of *histochemistry*—which literally means "chemistry of cells." Histochemistry is now a widely used technique to localize and visualize cellular components under the microscope using different stains. The technique is an essential constituent of biomedical and pathological research and is utilized for the diagnosis of many diseases, including cancer and Alzheimer's disease. Bourne later studied the healing process for wounds and the localization of enzymes in hard and soft tissues. Among his most important books are *Structure and Function of Muscle* (1962) and *Biochemistry and Physiology of Bone* (1956). His works on primatology include *Ape People* (1970), *Primate Odyssey* (1974), and *The Gentle Giants: The Gorilla Story* (1975).

Karl Landsteiner (1868–1943) an Austrian-born American who began his career in 1897 as an assistant in pathological anatomy at the Institute of Pathological Anatomy in Vienna. Over ten years, he performed nearly 4000 post-mortem anatomical examinations and published about seventy-five articles on his observations of blood chemistry. In 1911, he became an associate professor of pathological anatomy at Vienna University where he published on anatomy, bacteriology, histology, and virology. In 1922, he emigrated to New York and worked at the Rockefeller Institute. Landsteiner shifted his attention to the study of blood groups, which masked his anatomy accomplishments. He became much more famous for his blood work, which later won him a Nobel Prize (Chapter 9).

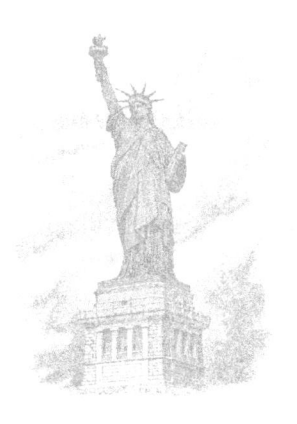

CHAPTER 3

American Medical Education and Educators

Doctors are teachers, whereas surgeons are those who work with their hands; that is the definition of the words. Doctor is a word derived from the Latin verb "docere," meaning to teach; the term was invented in Middle Ages to designate eminent scholars. Although some specialists—such as dentists, chiropractors, and podiatrists—also use the title doctor, the *Canadian Press Stylebook* decrees that only physicians should be called doctors. The Ph.D. or Doctor of Philosophy generally uses the title doctor. The word 'surgeon' comes from the Greek *kheirourgos*, meaning "done by hand" and designated for those who use their hands for surgery. Surgeons study medicine and become physicians before receiving surgical training. Physicians (who include surgeons) are teachers to their patients—though some have academic positions in medical schools, universities, and teaching hospitals and are also involved in the education of medical students, residents, and fellows.

Before the American Revolution, formal medical training did not exist. Practitioners were trained chiefly through apprenticeship; only a few ambitious practitioners could afford the time and expense to travel abroad for further education at a school or hospital. In colonial times, America, as in Europe, had more surgeons than doctors. Surgery was not viewed as belonging to the same sphere of medical treatments until 1745, when English barbers and surgeons finally parted ways. By the 19th century, training had become unified so that surgeons and physicians went through the same medical schools. Colonial Americans, during the 1600s and first half of the 1700s, who hoped to become physicians did so by apprenticing themselves to an established physician who may have trained in Europe. Some named themselves doctors, without any training, by establishing a reputation as a medic treating patients or selling therapeutics.

This incensed one colonial physician who spoke out against pseudo-practitioners and advocate for official medical training for physicians. His name is **William Douglass**, and he was born in Gifford, Scotland. He received his medical degree in 1712 from the Netherlands. Douglass came to the US in 1716, settling in Massachusetts Bay Colony and practicing in Boston. He authored a proposal in 1737, calling to register all medical practitioners in the Province of Massachusetts Bay. This made him unpopular among fellow physicians (Chapter 4).

The middle of the 18th century witnessed a change in American medical education when educators began to feel the need to establish institutions to train students to become doctors. Medical colleges were founded in Pennsylvania, New York, Boston, New Hampshire, and Baltimore.

John Morgan was an American physician and son of Welsh immigrants, who received his medical Education in Edinburgh, Scotland (a prominent medical education center). Morgan perceived the need for combining classroom teaching with bedside instruction in educating new physicians. William Shippen Jr studied medicine with his father and was also an Edinburgh-trained physician who upon return to Colonial America commenced America's first series of anatomy lectures in 1762. William Harrison, the ninth president of the US, briefly studied medicine at the University of Pennsylvania under William Shippen Sr and Benjamin Rush. Morgan and Shippen Jr would later found the first medical school in North America, the College of Philadelphia, which is today the University of Pennsylvania. Morgan and Shippen later became adversaries.

The Medical College of Philadelphia offered two degrees, a Bachelor of Medicine and a Doctor of Medicine. A bachelor's degree student took one course of lectures including anatomy, attended clinical practice in Pennsylvania Hospital for one year, served an apprenticeship to a reputable physician, and passed a public examination. For a doctorate, a student had to possess a bachelor's degree in medicine for three years and then write and publicly defend a thesis. Yet the model for most American medical schools' education was privately operated and lacked national oversight.

Other medical schools would be soon to follow. Columbia University was established in New York City in 1767, Harvard medical school in 1783, and Dartmouth School of Medicine in 1797. In 1807, the University of Maryland would be established by physicians as a private venture. By 1820, there were about 13 medical schools in the US. With expanding population, many physicians acquired training by apprenticeship, rather than going to medical schools. In the latter part of the 19th century, some medical schools began to raise their entrance requirements. The founding of Johns Hopkins medical school in 1893 brought two events that drastically reshaped American medical education, establishing a medical association and a new model of medical training.

Johns Hopkins (1795–1873) was a Baltimore merchant and banker who became a philanthropist. As a youngster he worked in tobacco fields and later became a successful tobacco and alcohol merchant. His wealth multiplied through his stocks in the railroad. He gave $1 million to build a children's orphanage. In 1867, he made a donation to build the university and hospital that carry his name. When he died his worth was $8 million, and $7 million of this went to the university and hospital; this was the largest philanthropic bequest in US history. In his will, he wanted the hospital to treat the homeless of Baltimore pro bono. It took 16 years for Johns Hopkins Hospital to be built—and 20 years for the university. Johns Hopkins was literally a hospital on a hill, located at 601 North Broadway. It opened as part of the university in May 1889, with a bust of Johns Hopkins in the rotunda and 600 people attended the festivities.

The American Medical Association (AMA) was established in 1847 because of some physicians' concerns with the quality of US medical education, as well as medical fraud and unscientific practices. One of these concerned physicians was Nathan Davis, who while in Binghamton, NY, obtained a cadaver and demonstrated anatomy to medical students. Initially, he was teacher, lecturer, and demonstrator of anatomy at the College of Physicians and Surgeons in New York City. Later, he became central in establishing the AMA, serving as its president twice and the first editor of its Journal. The AMA established the world's first code for ethical practice in medicine to improve physicians' low public image and advocated for medical education of physicians and research, exposing quack remedies. Today, the AMA is one of the largest medical societies in the world.

In 1900, US medical school education was informal, admissions standards were low, and sometimes the only requirement was a high school education, which resulted in ill-prepared physicians. In the beginning of the 20th century, a group of men, disillusioned by the poorly trained physicians in American medical schools, formed the Hopkins Circle at Johns Hopkins University and launched an initiative to improve the sorry state of medical education in America. The group comprised William Welch, a pathologist and dean at Hopkins,

William Osler, an internist and pathologist, and Frederick Gates, a Baptist minister. The group invited a former schoolteacher, Abraham Flexner, to survey the quality of medical schools throughout America and Canada and provide suggestions for their improvement.

Flexner had studied classics at Johns Hopkins University and then psychology at Harvard University and University of Berlin. He taught Latin and Greek in Louisville and devoted much of his life to education. He modeled his educational philosophy on that of John Dewey, the progressive who advocated learning by doing and solving problems, rather than rote learning.

Using Johns Hopkins as the gold standard for all other schools in the survey, Flexner was guided by the German model of medical education as the prototype, which deemed science as the main dynamism in shaping the ideal physician. Flexner sought the advice of members of the AMA Committee and the Carnegie Foundation, which sponsored the study. Flexner's 374-page report was a damning indictment that described nearly all medical schools as defective in at least one of many criteria—including low admission standards, poor laboratory facilities, and minimal exposure to clinical material. Many were proprietary schools running for profit. Flexner report found that 50 of 155 schools were associated with universities, but only two Johns Hopkins and Harvard required a 4-year college degree for admission, while others required a year or two—some, none at all.

Flexner recommended at least two years of prior college or university study, as a requirement for admission and suggested medical education should last 4 years; two on basic sciences and two on clinical studies. The critique of medical education included in the Flexner Report of 1910, and its recommendations would transform the nature and process of medical education in America, eliminating proprietary schools and establishing the academic biomedical model as the gold standard of medical training. Twenty years after the report's publication, the original 131 medical schools had reduced to 76. One of the new paradigm shifts was hiring full-time faculty professors to medical schools. The group's efforts and Flexner report resulted in the modern science-based foundation of medical training in the US, which is recognized today as a leader in medical education and research.

In 1928, the Medical College Admission Test (MCAT) was developed as a requirement for admission to medical schools. Today most medical school graduates engage in one of 135 residency training specialties averaging five years and vary from three to seven years. After residency training, many specialists also seek a one-year fellowship to gain in-depth expertise in one field. After completion of all medical education, physicians in practice are required by medical specialty boards to maintain their certification. This is accomplished through continuing medical education and passing periodic examinations.

Today, there is more to educating physicians than continuing medical education and lifelong learning of scientific material. Non-medical skills are advocated by medical and surgical organizations to their member physicians. These aptitudes include patient advocacy, communication, and empathy. Patient-centered care is the new paradigm shift away from disease-centered care. Leadership, ethics, and professional responsibility are paramount for physicians to regain some of the trust that has been eroded lately between physicians and patients. Physicians conducting medical research are now adhering to guidelines that safeguard against any biased results that pose maleficence to patients and ensure the resolution of any conflict of interest doctors may have. The Hippocratic oath includes the promise to abstain from doing harm to patients. During World War II, Nazi medical war crimes were committed when physicians conducted painful and deadly experiments on prisoners without their permission. At the Nuremberg war crimes tribunal of 1946, sixteen physicians were found guilty, and seven were sentenced to death. The Nuremberg code listed a set of ethical research principles for human experimentation and stressed the absolute need for voluntary consent of human subjects. Physicians, while practicing

21st-century medicine face a number of challenges. Despite barriers, doctors continue to provide exemplary care, largely thanks to the efforts of medical educators over the last 100 years.

A subset of medical doctors is considered *physician-scientists* because they seek further knowledge by setting aside time besides clinical practice to conduct research. As a result, some have made scientific breakthroughs that significantly reduce or eradicate disease. Although physician-scientists now represent about 2% of physicians, more than half of the Nobel Prize laureates in physiology and medicine are physicians engaged in scientific research. The growing complexity and specialization of medical sciences and healthcare delivery have recently compelled physicians to seek further formal training in research and acquire an additional Ph.D. degree or engage in an MD/Ph.D. program, thus dedicating substantial time out of their career for scientific investigation. The American Physician Scientists Association was established in 2003 to address the needs of these physician-scientists in regard to training and career development.

Osteopathic medicine is a field of healthcare that emphasizes the role of the musculoskeletal system in disease prevention and treatment. It began in response to the frequently harmful American medicine being practiced in the 1800s. Osteopathy was originally based on the philosophy that most disease is due to mechanical interference of nerves and blood flow, which can be cured by realigning bones, nerves, and muscles. Andrew Still was an army surgeon who established the American School of Osteopathy in Kirksville, Missouri in 1892. His motive was the poor practices of the conventional medical system that lacked credible efficacy and was morally corrupt. His intention was to introduce a rational medical therapy that would consist of the manipulation of the musculoskeletal system, surgery, and sparing use of drugs. He claimed that he could shake a child and prevent scarlet fever, croup, diphtheria, and whooping cough. Initially, he faced opposition from the medical establishment, including the AMA. Later, the profession transformed itself; and today, graduates of osteopathic medical colleges are designated as Doctors of Osteopathic Medicine (DO). They are licensed to practice any domain of medicine and surgery, and most do not use manipulations in their work. Cranial Osteopathy involves skull manipulation which—albeit controversial—continues to be utilized by a few practitioners. Although still called osteopathy, this term is now designated to the practice outside the US, where the discipline was exported to European and Commonwealth nations; these osteopath's training focuses on musculoskeletal manipulative techniques, and they are not licensed to prescribe medications or perform surgeries.

Two health domains that do not require their specialists to graduate from medical school are chiropractic and podiatry. Chiropractic, which was discussed earlier, emphasizes the body's ability to heal itself. The immigrant Canadian **Daniel Palmer** arrived in the US in 1865 and practiced magnetic healing and spiritualism as an alternative to medicine. In 1897, he founded the Palmer School and Care, which was renamed Palmer College of Chiropractic. In 1906, Palmer was prosecuted under the new medical arts law in Iowa for practicing medicine without a license and was jailed briefly. Throughout its history, chiropractic has been a subject of controversy and criticism because many chiropractors still believe that joint subluxation is the sole cause of disease and that manipulation is the cure for all human diseases.

Podiatry is an ancient profession. Napoleon employed a podiatrist to treat pain in his small feet, probably caused by wearing tight boats reaching his calf. President Lincoln suffered greatly with his feet and chose an immigrant British-American chiropodist named **Isachar Zacharie**—who not only cared for the president's feet, but was also deployed by the President on secret missions to deliberate with leaders of the Confederacy during the Civil War. The first society of *chiropodists*, who are now known as *podiatrists*, was established in New York in 1895, whereas the first school of podiatry was opened in 1911. Although podiatrists do not graduate from medical schools and do not have an MD degree, their podiatry school curriculum has subjects necessary for treating certain conditions affecting the foot.

Immigrant Medical Educators

The American sisters of Lebanese descent, Louis and Selma DeBakey were professors of scientific communication at Baylor College of Medicine. They were pioneers in the field of biomedical communications and the first to create a niche teaching doctors to read, write, think critically, and articulate eloquent language. Between the 1940s and 1960s, through lectures and publications, the sisters improved the field of medical writing and editing for physicians by designing and teaching courses to help doctors improve their academic writing and relay clear and concise medical information to patients. Immigrant physicians from Europe played a key role in professionalizing medicine and enriching earlier medical education, in the US, across different disciplines and teaching institutions. Only those pioneer educators who were born in the 19th century or prior and made lasting contributions will be the subject of this segment.

Doctors are present at the most intimate moments of their patients' lives: at their birth, on passing and every moment between. Patients turn to physicians for answers, counsel, and wisdom on some of the most urgent or life-threatening conditions. Doctors often offer patients suitable treatments but sometimes do not have the right solutions for their problems. Communicating with patients is a skill that medical schools do not offer in their curriculum. A Canadian-born medical educator focused on this area of communication at Johns Hopkins medical school. His name was **William Osler** (1849-1919) and he was born in Bond Head, Canada (Ontario) and educated at Trinity College, where he developed a passion for natural sciences. Osler enrolled in the Toronto School of Medicine; there, he performed post-mortem examinations and developed an interest in pathology but ultimately received his medical degree from the McGill University Faculty of Medicine in

Montreal, where he became a professor. Osler created the first formal journal club, where groups of learners met regularly to critique articles in academic medical literature. The journal clubs endured and continue to this day to be utilized in medical training programs. During the Montreal years, Osler performed more than 900 autopsies, as well as making several visits to the US and later taking an interest in post-Civil War educational reforms through the Hopkins Circle and Flexner report.

In 1884, Osler **(Fig 9)** moved to the US and was appointed Chair of Clinical Medicine at the University of Pennsylvania. When he left Philadelphia in 1889, he gave a famous farewell address, "*Aequanimitas.*" Osler then became Physician-in-Chief of the new Johns Hopkins Hospital, and in 1893 was instrumental in creating the Johns Hopkins School of Medicine, serving as one of the school's first professors of medicine.

While in Baltimore, Osler published *The Principles and Practice of Medicine* (1892), a textbook that established him as the world's leading authority in teaching modern medicine. The book became an industry standard and was translated into French, German, Russian, Portuguese, Spanish, and Chinese.

Along with William Welch, William Halsted, and gynecologist Howard Kelly, Osler was one of the luminous "Big Four" founding professors of the Johns Hopkins Hospital who led the hospital to greatness. Osler and Halsted established the first formal residency-training program in the US for postgraduate medical specialized education. The program required residents to reside at the hospital and be available 24/7 on call. This concept spread across the English-speaking world and continues to

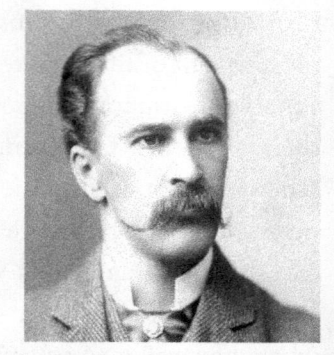

Fig 9. Canadian-born medical educator William Osler, one of the luminous "Big Four" founding professors of Johns Hopkins Hospital and author of famous essay *Aequanimitas*. (Wikipedia)

be implemented in teaching hospitals. In 1905, Osler left for England and became a Professor of Medicine at Oxford University, a position he held for fourteen years until his death. Osler was a founding donor of the *American Anthropometric Society*, a group of academics who vowed to donate their own brains for scientific study. Osler's brain was placed at the Wistar Institute in Philadelphia, and later held in the Mütter Museum in Philadelphia.

Osler was a true citizen of the world, Canadian by birth, an American expatriate, knighted as a baronet by King George V in 1911 in England. During his twenty-one years in the US, he made his most innovative and lasting influence on didactic medical education, bedside teaching, in ward rounds, and exemplary patient care. He believed that medical education should not be a business. Osler once said, "One of the first duties of the physician is to educate the masses." He believed that learning and teaching must go hand in hand and should be present at the patient's bedside. Osler's name was given to several diseases, medical signs, and symptoms, and more than a dozen buildings, schools, halls, and houses in various parts of the world.

Aequanimitas remains one of his most famous essays—the speech which Osler delivered to new doctors in 1889 as his farewell address at the Pennsylvania School of Medicine prior to his transfer to Johns Hopkins. In 1904, a book was published entitled *Aequanimitas with Other Addresses to Medical Students, Nurses, and Practitioners of Medicine*, which included 22 of the addresses that he gave. The book became a medical classic, and other editions were published. *Aequanimitas* espouses the serenity of mind, the calm amid the storm, and the equanimity and tolerance necessary for a physician's character. Today, the term emotional intelligence is an expansion of the same concept. *Aequanimitas* is the motto that sits on the Osler family crest and appears on the staff tie and scarf given to incoming interns at Johns Hopkins teaching hospital.

Osler was a paradigm of integrity and wisdom; few individuals had greater influence on American medicine and medical education than Osler. Besides the crucial role that Osler played in medical education, there are four other immigrant physicians who hold a special place in US medical education.

A medical dictionary is a lexicon of medical words developed for medical students, physicians, and researchers. *Stedman's Medical Dictionary* is the earliest of the three available dictionaries, which was published in 1833 by a British immigrant educator. This physician emigrated to the US on the request of President Thomas Jefferson and settled in Charlottesville to become an educator and full-time professor of medicine at the University of Virginia. He became well regarded and acted as personal physician to four presidents, including Thomas Jefferson, and was at Jefferson's bedside when he died. **Robley Dunglison** (1798–1869) was born in Keswick, England, and studied medicine in London, Edinburgh, Paris, and Germany. In 1818, he established a medical practice in London. In 1824, Thomas Jefferson offered Dunglison a professorship in anatomy and medicine. By 1825, Dunglison had joined the faculty of the University of Virginia where he became a full-time professor of medicine (Chapter 2).

Besides practicing medicine in Virginia, Dunglison developed an interest in anatomy and lexicography. Alongside his writing on anatomy and physiology, he published one of the earliest medical dictionaries, the *New Dictionary of Medical Science and Literature* (1833) which was the precursor of *Stedman's Medical Dictionary*. In 1903, Thomas Stedman became editor of the medical dictionary, making thorough revisions to the text and in 1911 publishing the dictionary that now carries his name. Currently, *Stedman's Medical Dictionary* is in its 28th Edition, which was published in 2005, and holds over 107,000 entries.

Dunglison **(Fig 10)** left the University of Virginia in 1833 for a professorship at the University of Maryland, but left Baltimore three years later, accepting a professorship at Jefferson Medical College, where he remained until his retirement; he served as dean of that college. In 1938, Dunglison became a naturalized US citizen.

Dunglison was a prominent medical educator and wrote *The Medical Student; or, Aids to the Study of Medicine* (1837). He published multiple medical books and was first to describe Huntington's disease in his textbook *The Practice of Medicine* (1842). In addition to Jefferson, Dunglison was also personal physician to Presidents James Madison, James Monroe, and Andrew Jackson.

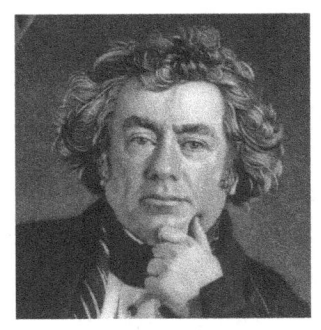

Fig 10. English-born immigrant Robley Dunglison medical educator, professor of anatomy and medicine Universities of Virginia and Maryland. Author of the dictionary that became known as Stedman's Medical Dictionary. (Wikipedia)

Two other important immigrant surgeons would come from the same homeland at the same period; one settled in New York and the other in Chicago. They both became educators and gifted their surgical expertise to their students and colleagues while offering care to patients in their communities. Besides lasting scholarly accomplishments that continue to benefit surgeons and patients today, they also possessed astonishing writing and artistic talents that have astounded the public until the present day. These two surgeons were **Arpad Gerster** (1848-1923) and **Max Thorek** (1880–1960).

Gerster was born in Kassa, Hungary (modern-day Czechoslovakia) and took a degree in medicine from the University of Vienna in 1872. Encouraged by his uncle who lived in New York, Gerster emigrated to the US in 1873 and began a general practice in Brooklyn. He received an assistant surgeon appointment at the German Hospital (Lenox Hill) in 1878, and later, the Mount Sinai Hospital. He gradually built a successful academic career and became the chair and professor of surgery at the New York Polyclinic. He espoused Lister's new antiseptic technique and became a distinguished teacher; among his pupils were brothers William and Charles Mayo. Gerster was the first to publish a textbook on the new technique in the US, *Rules of Aseptic and Antiseptic Surgery* (1888). In 1917, he published a popular autobiography entitled *Recollections of a New York Surgeon*. Besides being a physician, Gerster was also a linguist, musician, sketch artist, traveler, naturalist, and writer with an extraordinary power of observation that is exemplified by diaries recounting his visits to the Adirondacks Mountains of New York.

Thorek was born in Northern Hungry, part of the Austro-Hungarian Monarchy (modern-day Slovakia) and emigrated to Chicago in 1897. He received a medical degree from Rush Medical College in 1904 and began a modest practice in one of Chicago's poor immigrant neighborhoods. He gradually excelled and established the Thorek Memorial Hospital, which is still in operation in Chicago's uptown neighborhood.

Thorek practiced obstetrics and general surgery and was one of the first to practice plastic surgery. Besides modernizing surgery, he is best known for founding the International College of Surgeons in 1935, which is a global organization dedicated to promoting excellence in teaching and practice for surgeons and surgical specialists worldwide. It works with various bodies, including the World Health Organization and the United Nations, through collaborative projects. The International College of Surgeons operates the International Museum of Surgical Science in Chicago, which was also established by Thorek in 1954. Thorek became an internationally acclaimed amateur photographer during the "pictorialist" movement with work sold at auctions. He authored several photography books including *Camera Art as a Means of Self-Expression* (1947) and *Creative Camera Art* (1937), writing an autobiography in 1943, entitled *A Surgeon's World*.

Thorek's son, Philip, became a distinguished general surgeon and teacher in his own right and wrote several scientific books that continue to be taught today. While in surgical training, I read Philip Thorek's anatomy and clinical diagnosis books.

Dutch-born **Isidore Snapper** (1889–1973) earned his medical degree from the University of Amsterdam in 1911. He developed an interest in medical education and explored the relationships between physiological research and clinical medicine; the subject of his thesis. In 1938, he emigrated to the US where he spent the rest of his long professional career; first, as medical advisor to the Department of War in Washington, DC; and later, in Mt. Sinai Hospital in New York City, the Cook County Hospital in Chicago, and finally, at Beth-El Hospital in Brooklyn.

Besides clinical research, Snapper shared his insights with the medical community in a landmark publication entitled *Meditations on Medicine and Medical Education: Past and Present* (1956). The book made a plea for teachers at US medical schools to retain an element of virtue and healthy respect during bedside teaching, stressing the value of didactic presentations from clinicians to offer ripe wisdom to learners.

Snapper was also widely admired for his great scholarly knowledge and clinical skill. While on a visit to China he conducted research that was published in 1941, on heart disease prevalence contrasting Chinese with Westerners in relation to diet, emphasizing prevention and protection from disease through plant-based foods and enhanced intake of linolenic acid, which belongs to the omega-3 fatty acids.

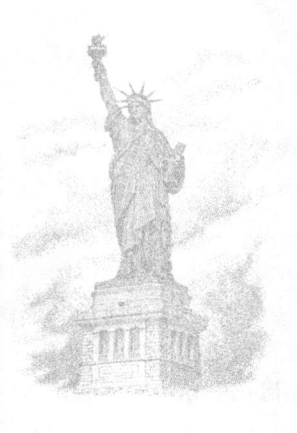

CHAPTER 4

Colonial and Revolutionary War Physicians

Immigrant Colonial Physicians

The American Revolutionary War was the first historic moment to truly push the limits of the country's physicians. To understand how this period would play out, we first need to consider the circumstances leading up to the War. The colonial era had begun with the colonization of North America by Europeans in the early 17th century and continued until the incorporation of the thirteen colonies into the United States of America. 'Heroic medicine' was a rigorous treatment of bloodletting, purging, and sweating to shock the body, a concept that had existed since Hippocrates' and Galen's times. Some of the widely used preparations for this archaic treatment were emetics, camphor, mercury, purgatives, opium, and potassium nitrate. The colonial medical system was based on the theory of humors and the imbalance of the four bodily fluids. This therapeutic model was embraced in America from the mid-1700s to the mid-1800s.

Hospitals at the time of the Revolutionary War were often makeshift tents or field hospitals sometimes set up in barns, churches, or public buildings. Due to a lack of sanitation and medicine being in short supply, soldiers often had a better chance of surviving the battle filed than the hospital. Medicine during the Revolutionary War offered symptomatic rather than curative therapies. The supply of drugs from Britain had now ceased; therefore, settlers turned to local flora and Native American remedies as alternatives to conventional medicines. The Continental Congress established laboratories and storehouses to serve the needs of the army. At times, Midwives would act as doctors, and 40% of all medics were women.

Before 1846 in US and Britain, elective surgeries were rare, and the most frequently performed operation was the amputation of a gangrenous limb, but the surgery itself often killed the patient due to subsequent infection. Surgeons used to perform surgeries in their own homes or in patients' homes. In 1809, American surgeon Ephraim McDowell successfully removed the first known ovarian tumor—weighing 22.5 pounds—through the abdomen without the benefit of anesthesia, antiseptic, or antibiotics onto his kitchen table. Before then, abdominal surgery was avoided for fear of fatal peritonitis—infection of the abdominal lining. It is difficult to imagine how bloody such surgery was without modern means of controlling bleeding, and it is likely that the patient and physician would be drenched in blood.

Some doctors of early colonial America were "ship surgeons" who did not have formal medical education. They were crossing the Atlantic from Britain and learned their trade through apprenticeship, gaining expertise by caring for travelers on the ships. As the colonies expanded and thrived, some earned medical degrees from universities abroad. Those few colonial physicians with formal degrees enjoyed greater status than apprenticeship physicians. On the eve of the Revolutionary War, there were an estimated 3,500 physicians in the colonies; about

400 of those had some informal training, and only about 200 actually held medical degrees.

Because 18th-century European medicine was advanced, some colonial physicians traveled to the medical school in Edinburgh, a destination attracting many students due to its reputation. Although doctors in the 19th century were better educated than their forerunners, study was not very sophisticated in the US, and there were few new discoveries that made much improvement to patient's care. However, throughout that century, American medicine began to improve slowly, all the while dependent on Western European physicians who began to emigrate to the US and brought with them many innovations and trends that continued for another two centuries.

The earliest immigrant physicians who came to the Promised Land during colonial and antebellum times were the founders of the republic's nascent medical field. Many of them were practicing not only medicine but religious doctrine as well.

The earliest known immigrant physician was **Samuel Fuller** (1580–1633), a British-born man who arrived in America on the *Mayflower*. Fuller came with his parents, who were Pilgrims from the separatist community in Leiden, Holland. His parents died in 1621, shortly after arrival, during the first winter. Fuller was a surgeon by trade but had sufficient education to practice medicine in the colonies. In 1629, Fuller visited Salem as a surgeon, but he was consulted by John Endicott, governor of the Massachusetts Bay Colony, about the practices of the Plymouth church. He then served as a church deacon and was appointed to settle disputes among the Indigenous people.

Fuller wrote about 30 books, mostly religious volumes but also medical books, dictionaries, and practical guides. He died among others in the Plymouth Colony during a smallpox epidemic. Fuller was indispensable as a self-educated physician, not only to those at the Plymouth colony but also to the surrounding areas of Salem and Charlestown.

In 1633, William Bradford also emigrated to Plymouth Colony on the *Mayflower*. In 1620, Bradford became a signatory to the Mayflower Compact and served as Governor of the Plymouth Colony. He commented on the epidemic that killed several colonists and specifically about Fuller's role stating, "In the end, after he had much helped others, Samuel Fuller who was their surgeon and physician and had been a great help and comfort unto them … being much missed after his death". The Pilgrim Hall Museum today holds the "Fuller cradle," which belonged to Samuel and his family's children, was constructed in Duxbury, and was made of maple and pine.

Two years before Fuller's passing, **Michael Wigglesworth** (1631–1705) was born in England, and at the age of seven, in 1638, his family moved to Charlestown, Massachusetts, later settling in New Haven, Connecticut. In 1651, Wigglesworth graduated from Harvard College and worked as a tutor; and, in 1654, he was appointed to the ministry in Malden, Massachusetts to be ordained.

Wigglesworth was a frail, small man plagued by poor health, which may have peaked his interest in medicine. In 1663, he went to Bermuda for seven months, where he studied medicine, eventually becoming a physician of the body and soul. His frailty often kept him from preaching in the pulpit, so he took to writing as a means of spreading the doctrine. He produced several poems, but his most celebrated literary work was the long religious ballad *The Day of Doom* (1662), which became America's first bestseller and a classic for a century after its publication. It was present in most New England Puritan households and sold 1,800 copies in its first year. The poem expounds the Puritan doctrines and offers a portrayal of the Day of Judgment and the damnation of the sinners. It was the longest poem in the Colonial Period, consisting of 224 stanzas. This may have played a role in indoctrination and the religious intolerance the Puritans would later adopt.

Wigglesworth was invited to join the Cambridge Association, a powerful group of ministers who solicited advice regarding witchcraft during the witchcraft trials of 1692. Wigglesworth attended some of their meetings but did not seem to have been an active participant. Wigglesworth left a lasting impression as a minister and poet, becoming a respected spiritual leader in his local community. Even after Puritan tenets began to abate across the country, his poems remained cited and studied.

The year Charles I declared war on his own Parliament, **Edward Taylor** (1642–1729) was born at Sketchley, Leicestershire, in England. Taylor grew up on a farm with a non-conformist family and later became a Protestant separatist. He worked as a schoolmaster at Bagworth village, but following the restoration of Charles II's monarchy, he refused to sign the 1662 Act of Uniformity that was implemented by the parliament, which cost him his teaching job. He began writing spiritual poems, lamenting the loss of religious freedom. His opposition to the Church of England and persecution at the hands of the clergy prompted him to emigrate to the Massachusetts Bay Colony in 1668. He later wrote a memoir about this Trans-Atlantic crossing and the first few years of his colonial life.

Shortly after arriving in Boston, he enrolled in Harvard College to study science and languages, but most importantly, medicine and ministry—all while taking a prestigious responsibility as a college butler. At Harvard, he roomed for two years with the British-born **Samuel Sewall**, who later wrote in criticism of slavery and became a Massachusetts Superior Court of Judicature. Taylor graduated in 1671 as a pastor and physician and accepted to serve in both diametrically opposite disciplines simultaneously at Westfield, in Western Massachusetts, where he stayed for the remainder of his life.

Although providing medical care was a major part of Taylor's career, there is no detailed account of his medical practice. This is partly because he was more driven by his religious fervor and most of what was written about him related to his religious writings and poems. However, we know Taylor did serve the medical needs of the city and the community beyond, as stated in a biographical essay, "Mr. Taylor discharged the duties of a physician, ministering alike to the bodily and spiritual wants of the population scattered over an extensive territory."

As a practitioner of medicine, Taylor was a follower of the Swiss physician, alchemist, and theologian Parcelsus—who popularized the view that observation must be combined with wisdom. This was evidenced by the books found in Taylor's library and the hand-written record of remedies he left in his dispensatory. These included botanicals modeled on the style of the English physician, botanist, and herbalist, Nicholas Culpepper. He also used animal tissue and even tissue derived from mummia—a medicinal preparation of mummified human flesh, which was a practice amongst physicians of Puritan New England. Shortly before that, in the 18th century, medical opinion began to turn against this practice.

Taylor would act as minister of the congregational church at Westfield for over 50 years. He became best known, however, as one of the earliest American Puritan poets and one of the foremost poets of that era. His immense corpus of poetry remained unpublished for nearly 200 years until a 7000-page manuscript was discovered in 1937. His two most important works are the *Preparatory Meditations* (1682–1725) and *Gods Determinations...* (1680). His poems were an expression of his deeply held religious views and the alarm by lapse of piety among his congregation; they also explore his struggle with some of the contradictions within the strict doctrine of Puritanism.

Another immigrant of the British Isles whose writings, advocating for hygienic practices in his community, were instrumental in establishing the field of public health and for becoming a state colonial governor. **Cadwallader Colden** (1688–1776) was born in Dunse, Ireland, to Scottish parents and a reverend father who wanted his son to become a cleric. Colden was sent to Edinburgh seminary school to become a minister. After graduation, Colden decided to visit London and study medicine, anatomy, and botany. After obtaining his medical degree, seeking better employment opportunities as a physician, he emigrated to Philadelphia in 1710, setting up a medical practice for the next seven years. He relocated to New York and became a surveyor general, which was the beginning of his political career but also the moment of his social and scientific accomplishments.

Colden **(Fig 11)** served as the first colonial representative to the Iroquois Confederacy: a group of Indigenous people from the Northeastern Woodlands and the Great Lakes of North America. This experience resulted in his *History of the Five Indian Nations* (1727), the very first book on the subject, where he discussed the religion, manners, customs, laws, and forms of government in this community—as well as battles, treaties, and trade of that group of tribes comprising the Mohawks, Oneidas, Onondagas, Cayugas, and Senecas.

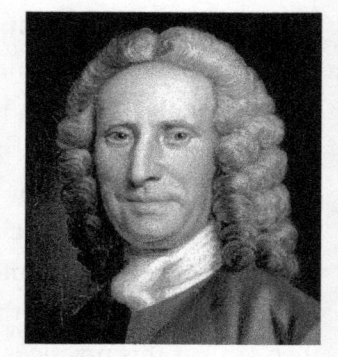

Fig 11. Irish-immigrant physician of the colonial period Cadwallader Colden was botanist, hygiene proponent, public health forefather, Natives advocate and acting governor of New York. (Public domain)

In 1739, Colden left New York City to live on a farm and dedicated much of his time to the scientific study of botany and the universe. Prompted by an epidemic of yellow fever, Colden published a series of essays on the correlation between unhygienic living conditions and high rates of disease in New York City in 1743. These essays were critical in establishing sanitation efforts in the city and established the field of public health. He also studied plant classification and wrote a taxonomy of flora near his home in Orange County, New York.

His political career was rekindled when he was elected to the provincial council, as lieutenant governor, and finally as acting governor of New York in 1760, a position he assumed on three further occasions. He defended the British Crown and was attacked by supporters of the Stamp Act. Like many politicians of his time, he was also a slave owner.

Colden's political career ended with his retirement from public life in 1775 when the British presence in New York ended at the start of the Revolutionary era. Colden died and was buried in a private cemetery in Spring Hill on Long Island in New York. Colden became a member of the Philosophical Society, an elementary school in Flushing, NY and a settlement in Montgomery, NY, were named in his honor

Another important colonial physician, who was discussed earlier, and friend of Colden was **William Douglass** (1691–1752). Born in Gifford, Scotland, he received his medical degree in 1712 from Utrecht University in the Netherlands. Douglass was a man far ahead of his time and one of the earliest colonial doctors to reject heroic medicine, speak out against pseudo-practitioners, and advocate for official medical training for physicians. This made him unpopular among fellow physicians.

Douglass first came to the US in 1716 and settled in Boston, where he remained until his death. Eventually, Douglass began to prosper in Boston and purchased property in the city and in Massachusetts Bay. He corresponded for 25 years with Colden about botany and medicine. As a result, Douglass accumulated a collection of 1,100 American plants.

Douglass was not popular in the Puritan community or among other physicians of the city. He joined the emerging dissenters against Puritanism in Boston. Although he was a skillful practitioner and member of the earliest medical society in America, he was disliked by other less qualified physicians; in 1721, he claimed he was the only physician in Boston with a medical degree. He criticized the prevailing system that allowed anyone with only a one-year apprenticeship with any practitioner to claim he was a physician. He blamed fellow physicians for their patients' deaths—as they often resorted to bloodletting or emetics as treatment for all diseases. He was probably the author of a proposal in 1737 calling for a register of all medical practitioners in the Province of Massachusetts Bay.

When a smallpox epidemic spread through Boston in 1721, Mather urged physicians to adopt the practice of inoculation in Boston. The other physicians, including Douglass, opposed the procedure because of safety concerns. This is when a fallout between these two men transpired. Douglass did not rush into practicing inoculation but consequently he became convinced that the inoculations were safe and effective; he later began to give inoculations.

Over two years, another epidemic of diphtheria and scarlet fever spread across Boston. Douglass wrote an account of the outbreak, *The Practical History of a New Epidemic Eruptive Miliary Fever, with an Angina Ulcusculosa, Which Prevailed in Boston, New England, in the Years 1735 and 1736*. This publication was a masterful clinical description and one of the most accurate essays on diphtheria. It is also the first adequate account of scarlet fever. Colden praised Douglass for describing the only successful method of curing the disease.

Besides his medical practice and writing pamphlets on medicine, Douglass also wrote on economics and politics. He condemned the use of paper money by the American colonies, an approach that attracted a favorable response from Adam Smith, who cited his work in *The Wealth of Nations*, calling him the "honest and downright Dr Douglass." Douglass also observed the weather and studied magnetism and astronomy. His early colonial almanac *Mercurius Novanglicanus* (1743) includes scientific discoveries of the time. His map of New England, which was published posthumously, became the basis for other maps of the region for the following fifty years. Following a substantial financial donation in 1746, the town of New Sherburn in Worcester County, Massachusetts, changed its name to Douglas in his honor.

Physicians, Politicians, and Patriots of the American Revolution

Physicians at the dawn of the American Revolution were called upon to treat injured settlers during skirmishes with the Redcoats. While practicing medicine and surgery in Boston, one Founding Father of the nation, Dr Joseph Warren, became a member of the Sons of Liberty. Warren conducted an autopsy on the body of eleven-year-old Christopher Seider, shot in 1770 by a loyalist and the first casualty of the American Revolution during the Boston Massacre.

Immigrant physicians of the Revolution served as war surgeons but sometimes also forsook their vocation to become politicians, state governors, or high-ranking military officers in the army. Nine physicians, politicians, and patriots of the Revolutionary period made particularly unique contributions to the struggle for Independence. Some were captured, imprisoned, and even tortured by the British. Below are the captivating stories of those nine individuals.

Historians know of **Matthew Thornton** (1714-1803) as a signer of the Declaration of Independence, but what many do not know is that he was also a very successful physician. Thornton was born near Derry, Ireland, and raised on a farm. In 1716, his family emigrated to Wiscasset, Maine, and settled in Worcester, Massachusetts, where he received a classical education. He pursued medical studies in Leicester, Massachusetts, through the time-honored tradition of apprentice study with an established physician—in his case, it was under the direction of a relative. In 1740, at the age of 26, he began what became a successful medical practice in the Scottish-Irish settler town of Londonderry, New Hampshire. He practiced for about ten years and became a distinguished physician and surgeon. In 1745, Thornton was appointed surgeon to the New Hampshire militia during King George's War (1745–1748) and participated in the expedition that captured Louisburg, the French fortress in Nova Scotia, in 1745. Thornton was praised by his superiors for his excellent medical skills; only six men in his entire regiment died of disease on this mission—an extremely low number for that time.

Thornton also engaged in local politics of New Hampshire, serving as president of its provisional congress and House of Representatives.

He was elected to the Continental Congress and later became the last to sign the Declaration of Independence document. Thornton was one of three signers of the Declaration of Independence who were originally born in Ireland—**James Smith**, and **George Taylor**, being the other two. He died and was buried in Thornton Cemetery in Merrimack, New Hampshire. A town in New Hampshire is named after him, along with an elementary school and US Route 3 in Merrimack.

William Irvine (1741-1804) was born to Scottish-Irish parents in Fermanagh, Ireland. After attending Trinity College in Dublin, he studied medicine under the renowned physician-anatomist George Cleghorn who would later vouch for Irvine's competency and knowledge of medicine. Irvine became a ship surgeon in the Royal Navy, serving at sea in the French and Indian Seven Years' War. Irvine emigrated to colonial America in 1763, settling in Carlisle, Pennsylvania.

When the Revolutionary War began, he raised the 6th Pennsylvania Regiment and became a colonel in the Revolutionary Army, later winning a promotion to brigadier general and serving under General George Washington. He participated in the invasion of Canada, was captured during the Battle of Three Rivers, and was imprisoned in Canada. After his release, he participated in the Battle of Monmouth and—for his service—was finally promoted to brigadier general in 1779 with command of the western frontier. In 1783, he was headquartered at Fort Pitt. With the support of Washington, Irvine helped neutralize the remaining British troops in Detroit. After the war, he became a statesman, serving in various posts while also practicing medicine. Finally, he served in both the Continental Congress (1787–88) and the US House of Representatives (1793–95) before taking on his final mission as a commissioner to resolve the dispute of the Whisky Rebellion.

In the latter part of his life, he helped found the Society of Cincinnati and became one of the six trustees of Dickenson College and superintendent of military stores, a position he held until his death in Philadelphia. The Town of Irvine bears his name, as well as a community in Warren County, Pennsylvania.

Edward Hand (1744-1802) was born in Clyduff, Ireland, received medical training at Trinity College, Dublin, and would become an army surgeon. In 1767, Hand enlisted as a Surgeon's Mate in the 18th (Royal Irish) Regiment of Foot. In the same year, he arrived with his regiment in Philadelphia and was stationed in Fort Pitt. In 1774, he resigned from his commission and returned to practice medicine in Lancaster, Pennsylvania, and decided to join the Freemasons. He helped establish a militia called the Lancaster County Associators. He later enrolled in the Continental Army, initially as a lieutenant colonel in the First Pennsylvania Regiment under Irish-American **William Thompson**. He was present during the struggle for Boston and New York, fighting at Trenton and Princeton. His regiment was crucial in delaying the British troops and preventing them from invading Manhattan's Throg Neck Peninsula. In 1777, he rose to the rank of Brigadier General, commanding Fort Pitt. Later, he was promoted to Brigadier Commander and Adjunct General in the Continental Army, working under the French General Marquis de Lafayette, where he saw action in battles such as the famous Siege of Yorktown, which ultimately ended the war. For his distinguished service, he was promoted to Brevet General. One of his tasks was to defend the western frontier against attacks by the Native Americans who were allied with the British and American Loyalists. One unfortunate event in his life history was his inability to distinguish the difference between separate Native American groups. Hand attacked the neutral Lenape natives in trying to reduce the Indian threat to settlers in the Ohio Country.

After the war, Hand returned to practicing medicine and was elected as a delegate to the Confederation Congress (1784–85), later becoming a member of the Pennsylvania Assembly and Pennsylvania Convention that ratified the Constitution. In 1791, President Washington appointed him inspector for revenue. He died a decade later and was interred in St James Episcopal Cemetery. A middle school in Lancaster was named after him; but in 2020, the parents voted to change the name because Hand had once taken ownership of a plantation that had one slave on it—thus, he was considered to be a slave owner.

There is one Irish physician of particular note for his contribution to US medicine, law, politics, and poetry—in addition to his gallantry on the battlefield. **Thomas Burke** (1747-1783) supported the Revolution and participated in the war in 1777, joining the army to battle advancing British troops. He became a lawyer and practiced both medicine and law but dedicated most of his time to being a politician. Burke was born in Galway, Ireland, and emigrated to Virginia in 1764 to settle in Norfolk and study medicine. He practiced medicine in Accomack County for several years but subsequently turned to law and became a practicing attorney. In 1772, he moved to Hillsboro, North Carolina, writing poems and essays and playing a prominent role in local politics. He served in the Provincial Congress and was later elected as delegate to the Continental Congress (1777–81), where he championed civil rights. In 1781, Burke was elected Governor of North Carolina. He was captured by Tories and imprisoned by the British on James Island, South Carolina. He managed to escape while under parole and resumed his duties as governor until 1782. His health never fully recovered from his mistreatment during imprisonment. A county became his namesake even before his serving as a governor.

David Jackson (1747–1801) was born in Newtown-Limavady, Ireland. After immigrating to the US around 1730, he attended the University of Pennsylvania and became a member of Pennsylvania's first medical school class, graduating with a degree in medicine in 1768. He first practiced medicine in Chester, Pennsylvania, before opening a practice in Philadelphia. He left Philadelphia only when the British troops occupied the city in 1777. Jackson volunteered on behalf of the Continental Congress to manage a lottery to raise funds for the Continental Army. He served as a field surgeon with the Pennsylvania militia for the entirety of the war. Later, he returned to Philadelphia to resume his medical practice and open an apothecary.

After the war, Jackson worked as an attending physician at Blockley Hospital for about three years. He then became a delegate to the Continental Congress in 1785. Subsequently, he left public service and ceased medical practice to concentrate on pharmacy. He introduced

what became known as 'David Jackson' recipes and 'home remedies.' Later, he served as a trustee of the University of Pennsylvania and was elected as a member of the American Philosophical Society in Philadelphia. Jackson died in Oxford, Pennsylvania.

Last but not least of the six Irish heroes was **James McHenry** (1753–1816) who grew up with a classical education in Dublin. In 1771, he emigrated to America and lived with a family friend in Philadelphia,

before finishing his preparatory education at Newark Academy (now University of Delaware). He studied medicine and, for two years was apprenticed under the renowned Philadelphia physician, Benjamin Rush, one of the signers of the Declaration of Independence. McHenry put his good training to the noble cause of his adopted country and volunteered his surgical services in a New York hospital, caring for the wounded, as well as medical departments in Massachusetts and Pennsylvania.

During the war, McHenry **(Fig 12)** was appointed as surgeon general in the Continental Army. He served with the Fifth Pennsylvania Battalion where he was stationed at Fort Washington. When the New York Fort fell to the British Army in late 1776, he was taken as a prisoner of war but released in a prisoner exchange, two years later. During captivity, he treated his wounded comrades and witnessed the poor medical care the prisoners were given—they

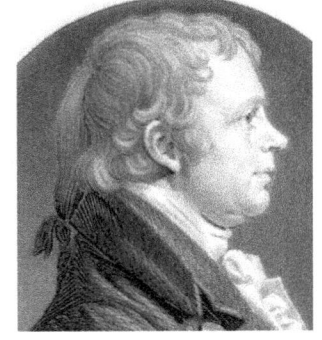

Fig 12. Irish-born James McHenry, Continental Army surgeon general, delegate to Continental Congress, and US Secretary of War. Fort McHenry is named after him. (Library of Congress)

were profoundly neglected by their captors. He briefed General George Washington on the abuse faced by these prisoners-of-war and wrote reports to that effect. He returned to duty and was assigned to Valley Forge, Pennsylvania, after which he was appointed to serve on General George Washington's headquarters staff as a secretary. During that period, he saw action in the battles of Monmouth and Springfield, New Jersey. Lastly, in 1780, he went to the service of the French General Marquis de Lafayette as a staff member and was granted the rank of major by the Continental Congress, until his retirement from the Army in 1781.

McHenry later entered politics. He was elected to the Maryland Senate—and also served in the Continental Congress. He campaigned for the Constitution in Maryland and attended its ratification. He then accepted Washington's offer in 1796 to take the post of Secretary of War and held it through Adams' administration. Because of his alignment with Alexander Hamilton and the Federalists, McHenry was forced to resign from his position as cabinet member in 1800. McHenry returned to his estate near Baltimore to semi-retirement. Baltimore's Fort Whetstone was renamed Fort McHenry in his honor and during the War of 1812, Fort McHenry became the birthplace of the US national anthem.

Two other physicians emigrated from the British Isles and a third from the Caribbean to become physicians, patriots, and politicians during the colonial period.

The first was a man whose name very much reflected his character. **Noble Wimberly Jones** (1723–1805) was English-born and a physician like his father, despite neither possessing formal education in the field. He emigrated to the colonies and settled in Savannah, Georgia in 1733. As a youth, he became a practicing physician for several years and served in the militia. He became a politician in Georgia and later a progressive civic leader who earned the title "Morning Star of Liberty" for his leading role in the colony's struggle for independence. He was taken hostage by the British and imprisoned in St Augustine, Florida. After the British occupation, he returned to Savannah and was elected as a delegate to the Continental Congress in 1781. Suffering a sword wound while quelling a mob, he resigned his position as speaker of the house and moved to Charleston, where he practiced medicine for the remainder of his life. Growing increasingly ill, Jones continued working until he died doing what he always aspired to do: serve his patients.

Few men can claim the astonishing and tragic military and political career of **Arthur St Clair** (1737–1818). Inheriting immense family wealth, the Scottish physician came to America and became one of the biggest landowners in western Pennsylvania, only to lose his fortune in service to his country. St Clair attended the famed University of Edinburgh medical school and was apprenticed to the renowned physician-anatomist William Hunter. He joined the British army in 1757 and came to America to serve in the French and Indian War.

St Clair settled in Ligonier Valley, Pennsylvania, and participated in community politics serving on the council and as county clerk. He settled a boundary dispute in 1774 and also diffused an army conflict between Pennsylvania and Virginia Colonies. He subsequently accepted a commission in the Continental Army as a colonel and was later promoted to Brigadier General, seeing action in Yorktown where the British surrendered to George Washington's army. After the war, St Clair was elected as a delegate to the Confederation Congress (1785–87). Delegates elected St Clair as President of the Congress, the only immigrant American to serve in that capacity.

After his presidency, General St Clair became governor of the Northwest Territory—including Ohio, Indiana, Illinois, Michigan, and parts of Wisconsin and Minnesota. St Clair is today considered a seminal Founding Father of the nation. In Ohio, a Fort, an avenue, two townships, and a city were named after him. In Pennsylvania, a hospital, four townships, a borough, and several counties were named in his honor. Alabama, Indiana, Illinois, Kentucky, and Missouri also have several places named St Clair.

Thomas Tudor Tucker (1745–1828) was born in Bermuda but studied medicine and received his medical degree from the Scottish University of Edinburgh. He emigrated to America in the 1760s and settled in Charleston, South Carolina, where he opened a medical practice. Tucker supported American independence and served in the South Carolina House of Representatives. In 1781, he joined the Continental Army as a hospital surgeon in the Southern Department where he served until 1783. Here, he played a vital role in supplying the rebel army with gunpowder stolen from a British base in Bermuda.

Tucker would be elected to the US House of Representatives and dispatched as a delegate to the Continental Congress where he served in the first two congresses (1789–93). Thomas Jefferson appointed Tucker treasurer of the United States, a position he held until his death—serving four presidents and establishing a record as the longest-serving US treasurer. Tucker was entrusted by President James Madison to be his personal physician. He died while in office in Washington, DC and is buried in the Congressional Cemetery.

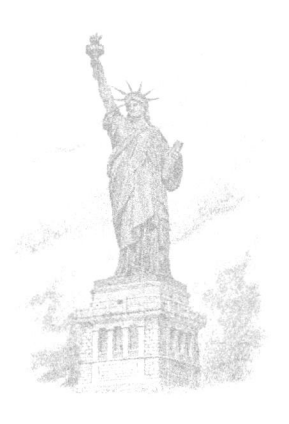

CHAPTER 5

Civil War Physicians

While the American Civil War was in full swing, European physicians and scientists had been learning about germ theory and antisepsis. This meant that by the time of the Civil War, doctors had better knowledge about hygiene. Despite this, battlefield surgery was still brutal, and sterile techniques remained foreign to the overwhelmed American physicians. Civil War doctors were tragically ill prepared; they did not specialize in war injuries and got their introduction to trauma surgery on the battlefield. They often operated in makeshift military hospitals and worked for 48 to 72 hours without sleep. Neither side of the conflict envisioned the scope of the horror that was about to be inflicted on them and the nation. Physicians could not cope with the massive number of casualties of the bloodiest war known to this country. On average, 430 soldiers died daily; and by the war's end, there were 1.7 million casualties in combat on both sides—a total of 630,000 deaths. In one day during the Antietam Creek Battle, there were 23,000 casualties.

Soldiers were wounded by bullets, artillery shrapnel, sabers, bayonets, or cannon balls. The slow-moving Minie bullet used during that time caused catastrophic injuries such as shattered limbs. Most were bullet wounds that led soldiers to lose limbs—or later, their lives due to infection. Wounds in the chest or abdomen were instantly fatal. Anesthesia was in its infancy and often the only anesthetic was from a whisky bottle. Three quarters of the surgeries performed were limb amputations, typically done within ten minutes using rudimentary chloroform or ether. If chloroform or whisky were unavailable, amputation was done while the patient was restrained by several men. Skin flap amputation took longer to do than circular amputation, and the lower limb also took longer than the upper limb. In both cases, however, the knife cut through the skin and muscles, then a saw was used for the bone; vessels were ligated to stop bleeding and a cast was applied so the surgeon could move on to the next amputation.

Shortage of doctors during the war drove many brave women to volunteer, including nurse nuns who assisted physicians in caring for wounded soldiers. Before the war, there were 113 doctors in the army; but by the end of the war, there were over 12,000 doctors in the Union Army—and over 3000 in the Confederate Army. As a result of the work of those dedicated surgeons on both sides of the conflict, they built up enormous experience in treating war-related injuries. Besides combat wounds, physicians had responsibility for caring for soldiers affected by illness. Challenges included overcrowded quarters and unhygienic camps, with contaminated water and spoiled food resulting in dysentery and cholera outbreaks. Yellow fever was a major problem, especially in the South. For every soldier who died in battle, two died of disease; among the illnesses involved were malaria, measles, smallpox, and typhoid fever.

Some Confederate army surgeons were slaveholders. However, immigrant physicians typically served in the Union Army and were for the most part abolitionists. We do not know how many Civil War physicians were immigrants, but we do know the stories of a few. There was no wartime correspondence, and detailed information on many of them is lacking. However, the majority of them came from Europe—particularly Germany and Ireland, as well as other locations.

Canadian Volunteer Physicians

Foreign-born physicians volunteered to serve in the Civil War; these were not necessarily immigrants as they returned to their countries after the war. We know of two who were Canadian citizens.

Robert Carrall (1837–1879) was born near Woodstock, Upper Canada and received his medical degree from McGill University in 1859. He practiced in Canada before becoming an assistant surgeon for the Union Army during the Civil War. He was on duty working in Emory and Henry College Hospital (1862–63) in Virginia and at the Marine US General Hospital, New Orleans (1863–65). After the war Carrall returned to Canada and became a politician for the remainder of his career. One of his accomplishments was a legislative bill he introduced to make July 1 a public holiday—to be called Dominion Day, and it is now called Canada Day.

Canadian Anderson Abbott (1837–1913) was born in Toronto to American parents of African ancestry who had fled Alabama after threats their store would be ransacked. His family became successful real estate Canadians. In 1858, Abbott became a medical student at the Toronto School of Medicine and became the first Canadian-born Black physician in 1861. During the Civil War, Abbott applied for a commission as an assistant surgeon in the Union Army but was refused. He reapplied as a medical cadet in the US Colored Troops, an all-black regiment, and was subsequently hired as a civilian surgeon. Abbott served in several US hospitals, including Freedmen's Hospital, which became part of Howard University. In 1865, he was assigned to a hospital in Arlington, Virginia.

Abbott was one of thirteen black surgeons to serve in the Civil War. He fostered a friendly relationship with President Abraham Lincoln and was in attendance when Lincoln was shot in April 1865. His widow, Mary Lincoln, later presented Abbott with a plaid shawl for his attempt to save the President's life.

After the war, Abbott returned to Canada and continued to practice medicine in Ontario, fighting against racially segregated schools. He then returned briefly in 1894, to be appointed surgeon-in-chief at Provident Hospital in Chicago, the first training hospital for Black nurses in the US—becoming the hospital's medical superintendent. Abbott resumed his private practice in Canada and also wrote. Publishing his work in *The Colored American Magazine* of Boston and New York, the *Anglo-American Magazine of London*, and *New York Age*. Medicine, biology, black history, the Civil War, Darwinism, and poetry were among his topics. Abbott was appointed aide-de-camp on the Staff of the Commanding Officers of New York, the highest military honor bestowed on a black person in Canada or the US. Abbott died in Toronto in 1913.

Canadian Immigrant Physicians

We also know of three Canadian-born American physicians who became Union army surgeons during the Civil War. One of those happened to become a physician consultant to the Confederate President Jefferson Davis. **Peter Pineo** (1825–1891) was born in Nova Scotia where he studied medicine but graduated in 1847 from Bowdoin Maine after a year at Harvard Medical School. He practiced medicine in various cities in Massachusetts and became a professor at the Castleton Vermont Medical College.

During the war, in 1861, Pineo was commissioned as Surgeon to the 9th Massachusetts Infantry—and later, appointed Brigade Surgeon of US volunteers. He was on the staff of Major General George Meade as Medical Director for the First Army Corps at battles in Antietam and South Mountain. He was ordered to Washington DC to command the US Douglas General Hospital, where he worked for the rest of the War. Pineo was promoted to Lieutenant Colonel in 1863 by President Lincoln and became Medical Inspector. When Confederate president Jefferson Davis was a prisoner at Fortress Monroe, Pineo was his consulting surgeon. After the War, Pineo led the US Marine Hospital Service at Hyannis, Massachusetts until his retirement in 1880. His Boston house purchased in 1850 is now the Phinney–Pineo House, owned by Barnstable Historical Society.

There is little record of the life and accomplishments of two Canadian-born physicians of the Union Army; **Samuel Ferrin** (1831-1875) and **Prosper Ellsworth** (1838–1907).

Ferrin was born in Saint-Thomas, Quebec, came to Wisconsin in 1857, graduated from Rush Medical College and practiced medicine and surgery in Darlington and Wingville Wisconsin. He first entered the military service as a private in Company I, 32nd Wisconsin. He then was enlisted as Union Army surgeon with the 32nd Wisconsin Infantry Regiment. He was commissioned First Assistant Surgeon of the 44th Wisconsin Infantry Regiment. In 1864, he was listed for duty at the post hospital in Nashville, Tennessee, where he remained until the end of the war. Besides a military career Ferrin while in Wingville became a highly esteemed member of the Third Assembly District during the 1872 session. Ferrin is buried in Union Grave Cemetery in Darlington Wisconsin.

We know much about **Ellsworth's** wife and the legacies both left behind. Ellsworth was born in Massawippi, Quebec. After moving to the US, he graduated from Rush Medical College, Chicago. During the war he became a Union Army surgeon as a major in the 106th Illinois Volunteer Infantry. After the war, in 1866, he established a medical practice in the spa city of Hot Springs, Arkansas. He was an organizer and the first Secretary of the Hot Springs Medical Society. In 1873, he married Sarah Van Patten a community activist founding a city library and established the Arkansas Federation of Women's Clubs in 1897. Doctor Ellsworth died in Hot Springs and was buried in Hollywood

Cemetery in Hot Springs. His cousin, Elmer Ellsworth, had been the first Union officer to die in the American Civil War. He was killed while removing a Confederate flag from the roof of the Marshall House Inn in Alexandria, Virginia.

The Ellsworth home in Hot Springs, known as "Wildwood House" was built in 1884 with Sarah Ellsworth's brother as architect, and was listed on the National Register of Historic Places in 1976. The house is now a bed and breakfast inn. The patriotic Sand Art Bottle, made by Andrew Clemens (1885-90) was presented to Ellsworth, featuring an eagle, flag, and medicine cup with pestle—it shows a dedication to Dr Prosper Harvey Ellsworth "From Two Friends". It was decorated with geometric and abstract designs throughout.

German-Born Immigrant Physicians

Up to one third of the Union Army soldiers were foreign-born, and many were children of immigrants—only a few thousand foreigners served in the Confederate Army. Thus, the Civil War came down to immigrants, and it was immigrants who won the Civil War. Most immigrant soldiers were Europeans, and Germans were by far the largest ethnic group, comprising more than 200,000 troops plus 250,000 second-generation immigrants. Some of these Germans were revolutionaries and had participated in a series of uprisings in Germany known as the 1848 Revolutions; they escaped persecution and emigrated to the US. Some of them came as physicians, while others studied medicine in the US.

We know of three German immigrant surgeons who served in the Union Army but not much is known about their upbringing, they are **William Goehrig** (1832-1903), **Louis Braun** (1825-1880) and **Charles Lehlbach** (1835-1895). However we have more information about eight other immigrant German physicians, seven of them served in the Union Army, some provided civic service to their communities and others introduced new rehabilitation methods that helped veteran soldiers.

William Wagner (1825–1872) was born in Karlsruhe and participated in the 1848 Revolutions, alongside compatriots **Carl Schurz** and **Franz Sigel**. In 1849, he escaped to Chicago where he established a medical practice. He served as an Army Major and surgeon in the 24th Illinois Infantry Regiment (1861–1863). Later, he became active in Chicago politics, serving as Coroner of Cook County, managing the Cook County Hospital (1866) and joining the Board of Health (1867). He married Matilda Brentano, daughter of fellow German immigrant revolutionary **Lorenz Brentano**.

Ernst Schmidt (1830–1900) was born in Bavaria and studied medicine at several universities, graduating in 1852 from Wurzburg. He became staff at Wurzburg Hospital and took a role in the failed German revolution, forcing him to immigrate in 1857 to Chicago. Here, he became an organizer and vice-president of the German Medical Society. In 1860, he was appointed to Humboldt Medical College in St Louis. He then served as a surgeon and major in 2nd Missouri Infantry Regiment. He resigned from the military when he became disabled. He was elected Coroner of Cook County (1862–1864). In 1867, he was on the staff of the Alexian Brothers Hospital and helped organize the first Jewish hospital in Chicago in 1869. In the 1879 Chicago mayoral election, Schmidt ran unsuccessfully for the Socialist Labor Party. Schmidt was also a scholar and translator of classical literature from Latin and Greek. He is buried in Chicago.

Mark Blumenthal (1831–1921) was born in Bavaria, immigrating to America with his parents in 1839 and growing up in Philadelphia. He graduated with a medical degree from Columbia University in New York City in 1852. He served as assistant physician in Blackwell's Island Hospital and deputy coroner of New York City in 1853. He visited Europe and worked as an attending physician in London, Paris, and Munich. Returning to America in 1854, he was appointed attending physician at the Jewish Hospital (Mount Sinai) until 1859.

When war broke out, Blumenthal served in the Third Regiment of the New York National Guard with the rank of Surgeon Major. He afterward became president and chief physician of the Institution for the Improved Instruction of Deaf Mutes, a Jewish facility where he created a new system to teach lip-reading to patients. Blumenthal was a founder of the Young Men's Hebrew Association, president of the Sabbath Observance Society of New York, president of the Jewish Chautauqua, and a trustee of the Congregation Shearith Israel.

Francis Huebschmann (1817–1880) was born in Riethnordhausen and graduated in medicine at Jena in 1841. He emigrated to the US in 1842 and settled in Milwaukee Wisconsin as the first German physician in the city, where he resided until his death. Huebschmann became a civic leader and played a leading role in Democratic state politics, serving as school commissioner (1843–51), member of the first Wisconsin Constitutional Convention (1846) and the committee on suffrage. He championed a provision in the constitution granting foreigners equal rights to Americans. He was a member of the Milwaukee City Council, a Milwaukee County supervisor, and Wisconsin State Senator (1851–62). He was also employed as superintendent of the affairs of the Native Americans of the Northern US (1853–57).

During the Civil War, Huebschmann resigned from politics temporarily and joined the Union Army in 1862 as surgeon of the 26th Wisconsin Infantry Regiment. He oversaw a division at the Battle of Chancellorsville and of the XI Corps at Gettysburg, where the Confederates held him captive for three days. He was also at the Battle of Chattanooga, ran the Corps hospital in Lookout Valley, and became brigade surgeon in the Atlanta Campaign. He was honorably discharged, and after the war, he returned to Milwaukee politics again to become state senator (1871-72), identifying with all the political, social, and musical activities of the German community. Lastly, he became affiliated with the US General Hospital. His remains are rested in Forest Home Cemetery, Milwaukee.

Henry Eversman (1837–1903) was born in the town of Iburg, Lower Saxony. His father first emigrated to America in 1835, returning to Germany to bring his family with him in 1845. Eversman attended city schools in Cincinnati. At age sixteen, he began teaching school in Teutopolis for a few years. Influenced by his physician father he studied medicine at Ohio Medical College in Cincinnati, graduating from that institution in 1861. In 1862, he was appointed by President Lincoln as Assistant Surgeon of Volunteers, and later was promoted to the rank of Surgeon and managed the army hospital in New Haven, Kentucky. In 1864, he was chief medical officer at Johnson's Island, on Lake Erie, at the prison for rebel officers where 3500 officers of the Confederate army were incarcerated.

After the war, in 1865, Eversman went to Effingham and became a general merchant, and later moved into banking as a member of Eversman-Wood & Engbring, private bankers of Effingham. After working in merchandising and banking, he discontinued the practice of medicine, twice serving as Mayor of Effingham. He died and was buried in Saint Anthony Cemetery in Effingham County, Illinois.

Few physicians abandoned their medical profession to dedicate their entire life to become army officers. One of those who did was **Louis Blenker** (1812–1863) whose passion for the military career overtook caring for patients. Born in Germany, Blenker trained as a goldsmith, but at the wish of his parents, opened a wine trading business. He then enlisted in the cavalry regiment and afterward studied medicine in Munich. Rather than taking up the medical profession he rejoined the military in 1848, to become a colonel in a revolutionary militia fighting against Prussian troops. His wife, Elise, accompanied him on his many campaigns. When the Prussian troops entered the Electorate of the Palatinate, he fought several times in Baden, but after the revolution failed, he fled Germany for Switzerland, then the

US in 1849, where he settled on a farm in New York and ran a small business.

During the War, Blenker became a colonel in the Union Army and organized the 8th New York Volunteer Infantry Regiment. He participated in many battles, including Bull Run and Cross Keys. For his bravery, he was raised to the rank of Brigadier General of volunteers. There were numerous testimonies of his gallantry, courage, and organizational ability. But he was a subject of controversy and accused of looting by his troops, as well as being careless with supplies and financial irregularities. This ruined his career. He was mustered out of service in 1863 and died in the same year in poverty of injuries sustained while on his farm in Rockland County New York, after a fall from his horse. He is buried in Rockland Cemetery of Sparkill, Rockland County, New York. If he had practiced medicine rather than served in the army, he probably would have been proved more valuable to his new country and appreciated by his patients.

The following are the stories of two German-American war surgeons who became more known for their advocacy of convalescence and for introducing new rehabilitation methods than for their surgical careers. Their military service will be highlighted but their other contributions will be addressed later.

William Detmold (1808–1894) was born in Hanover where he received his medical degree, moving to the US in 1837. During the war he volunteered as a civilian surgeon in Virginia at the First Battle of Bull Run. He became interested in amputation and rehabilitation technology for war veterans and introduced a knife that could be used by hand amputees. Detmold became a professor of military surgery and hygiene at Columbia University. He wrote and lectured regularly on war injuries, especially gunshot wounds to different parts of the body. One of his important medical contributions was to introduce orthopedic surgery to the US. He published an article about orthopedic surgery as a specialty and the first book on the treatment of clubfoot. In

1884, he became founder and first president of the New York County Medical Association.

Simon Baruch (1840–1921) was born in Schwersenz, Prussia, which is in modern-day Poland, emigrating to South Carolina as an adolescent in 1855. Baruch worked as a bookkeeper before studying medicine in 1859. He attended lectures at the Medical College of the State of South Carolina and enrolled at the Medical College of Virginia in Richmond, where he received a medical degree in 1862.

Baruch became a surgeon during the War, serving in the Confederate Army as an assistant surgeon to the 3rd South Carolina Battalion in 1862; in the same year, he transferred to the 13th Mississippi Infantry Regiment, and became a surgeon. After the Confederate defeat at Gettysburg in July 1863, he stayed on to treat the wounded. He was imprisoned at Fort McHenry in Baltimore but returned to his unit later and eventually to the 13th Mississippi Regiment, where he served until the end of the war.

During the Reconstruction Era, Baruch practiced medicine in South Carolina where he advocated for child smallpox vaccination and authored a widely read pamphlet on bayonet wounds. Baruch went to New York City, where he worked for one year as an attending physician to the Medical Polyclinic in the Manhattan district, tending to patients with infections. He served as President of South Carolina State Medical Association. His advocacy of public bathhouses and hydrotherapy and his honors and awards will be discussed later (Chapter 6).

Irish-Born Immigrant Physicians

When Dr Jonathan Letterman was designated to the Army of the Potomac as Medical Director, he focused on removing the sick and wounded from the battlegrounds, enforcing sanitary measures, maintaining the health of soldiers, and providing medical supplies. The army was in desperate need of a reliable ambulance corps. In August 1862, 3000 wounded were left on the field for three days and 600 were left for a whole week. Ambulance drivers replaced civilians, picked the pockets of the wounded, stole alcohol from the medical supplies, and left the injured to die. Letterman drew up a plan for an Ambulance Corps that would transport wounded soldiers without delay and devised field hospitals that removed surgeons from specific regiments and assigned them to division hospitals. In 1862, Letterman established field hospital systems carefully designed to work with the Ambulance Corps and the supply chain. For his effort, he became known as the "Father of Battlefield Medicine."

During the Battle of Fredericksburg, this holistic approach saw its first opportunity and was praised by another Irish-born surgeon whose writings have earned him a certain fame. His name is **Charles O'Leary** (1861–1897), then Medical Director of the Sixth Corps, who wrote about Letterman's new system. The following are excerpts of what he mentioned in his official report after Fredericksburg: *"Being appointed Medical Director of the Sixth Corps a few days prior to the battle of Fredericksburg, December 13, 1862, I had the opportunity of putting in operation the Field-Hospital organization devised by the Medical Director of the Army, and witnessing its beneficial results. ... all the necessary appliances were on hand, and the arrangements necessary for the proper care of the wounded were as thorough and complete as I have ever seen in a civil hospital ...the wounded were brought without any delay or confusion to the hospitals of their respective divisions."*

Another testimony made by O'Leary at Chancellorsville and Marye's Heights described the system's efficiency: *"In the operations at the time of the battle of Chancellorsville in the following May, the Sixth Corps charged and took Marye's Heights behind the town of Fredericksburg... in less than half an hour we had over 800 wounded. Two hours after the engagement, such was the celerity and system with which the ambulances worked, the whole number of wounded were within the hospitals under the care of nurses."*

After arriving in the US, O'Leary had immediately enlisted as a Surgeon, commissioned by Volunteers Medical Staff (1861) and was appointed Medical Director of the Sixth Corps just days before the Battle of Fredericksburg (1862). He was promoted to Lt Colonel, leaving the armed forces in 1865. In his memoirs, Letterman wrote of his admiration for his corps of surgeons and his profound confidence in them. He gave much credit to the surgeons from civil life. In his publication *Medical Recollections of the Army of the Potomac*, he praised and commended them in soldierly terms, most especially the services of O'Leary.

We have limited knowledge of three Irish born immigrant surgeons who served in the Union Army, **Francis Burke** (1828-1906), **Patrick Heaney** (1830-1865) and **Edward Donnelly** (1822-1891. However we know more about five surgeons, three of them actually joined the fighting ranks.

One surgeon in the Union Army military ranks became renowned for developing a new ink that was used for printing paper currency. **Thomas Antisell** (1817–1893), who was born in Dublin, attended the Dublin School of Medicine, the Apothecaries' Hall of Ireland, and the Royal College of Surgeons in London, graduating from the latter with a medical degree in 1839. He studied chemistry and geology, then held a lectureship in botany at St Peter School of Medicine until 1848, finally becoming a member of the Royal Dublin Society in 1844. Appalled at the inhumane treatment of his countrymen and women by their British overlords, he joined the nationalist movement for Ireland's independence. Fearing sedition charges, he emigrated to New York in 1848, where he set up a clinic while lecturing in many US cities on medical topics—including military surgery.

When the war broke out, Antisell joined the Union Army as Brigade Surgeon of volunteers with the rank of major. His original assignment was to act as medical director with various Corps in the Army of the

Potomac, including the 12th Army Corps. In 1862, he was made chief surgeon at Harewood Hospital in Washington DC. He also served as president of a medical examining board and as surgeon in charge of sick and wounded officers in Washington DC. He eventually became a lieutenant colonel in 1865 and was honorably discharged with the rank of colonel. After the war, Antisell went to the Empire of Japan and worked as a chemist, where he developed inks for printing paper money. In the US, he then worked at the patent office and continued publishing on topics including chemistry, botany, oceanography, city sanitation, and animal disease. Antisell died in Washington DC and is buried in the Congressional Cemetery.

After German immigrants, the Irish were the largest contingent of foreign-born soldiers to fight in the Civil War: approaching 200,000. When Fort Sumter was attacked, the first casualty of the Civil War was an Irish private—**Daniel Hough**, when a gun misfired during the surrender and blew his arm off; he soon died of his injury. It is estimated that 30,000 Irish were killed during the war. One of these was a surgeon who was killed in action at the Battle of Cedar Creek. His name is **Joseph Thoburn** (1825–864) who was born in County Antrim in Northern Ireland. In 1826, his family moved to the US and settled on a farm near St Clairsville, Ohio. Thoburn taught at a school for several years before studying medicine at Starling Medical College in Columbus, Ohio. After graduation, he relocated in 1849 to Brownsville, Pennsylvania, where he briefly partnered in a medical practice before resigning to accept an appointment in Columbus at the Ohio Lunatic Asylum as an assistant to the chief physician. In 1853, he moved to Wheeling, Virginia where he established a successful private medical practice.

When the bombardment began in Charleston Harbor in April 1861, triggering the war, Thoburn **(Fig 13)** enlisted as surgeon to the 1st Virginia Infantry, and accompanied his regiment in the Battle of Philippi, where patients included his own wounded Colonel. After the regiment was placed out of service, most soldiers reenlisted in the 1st Virginia Infantry. Thoburn was commissioned as Colonel of that regiment. He commanded troops in several battles in West Virginia and Shenandoah Valley in 1862 and 1863. The following year, he assumed command of a division in the VIII Corps and fought in the Valley Campaigns of 1864 in the army of Philip Sheridan. He was wounded in 1862 in the First Battle of Kernstown, one of the rare defeats faced by Confederate General Stonewall Jackson, though Thoburn recuperated and rejoined the battle a month later. During the Battle of Opequon, Thoburn's division took a position at the edge of woods and ambushed troops to score a spectacular victory for the Union.

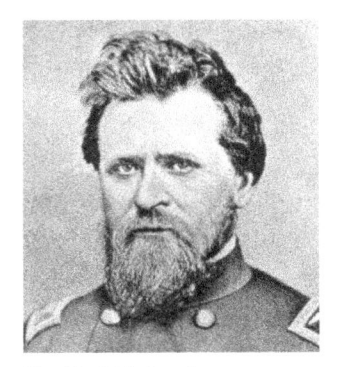

Fig 13. Irish-immigrant surgeon, Joseph Thoburn, while serving his adopted country was shot and killed during the Battle of Cedar Creek in Shenandoah Valley. (University of West Virginia)

On October 19, 1864, Thoburn was shot through his left side and killed in action during the Battle of Cedar Creek in Shenandoah Valley, which would become another Union victory. His corps commander, George Crook, reported, "*I am pained to report the death of Col. Joseph Thoburn, commanding First Division, and Captain Philip G. Bier, assistant adjutant-general on my staff. Both fell mortally wounded while rallying the men. Brave, efficient, and ever conspicuous for their gallantry on the field of battle, in them the country sustained a loss not easily repaired.*" A biographer later wrote, "*Dr. Thoburn was greatly beloved by his brother officers and men, as a man full of kindness and benevolence, and of undoubted bravery and patriotism. As a physician, he possessed very clever attainments, with a high sense of professional honor.*"

Thoburn's body was taken to Wheeling for a magnificent public funeral. It was taken with a military escort to Mt Wood Cemetery with a public procession including city officers, council, medical faculty, military escort, and many citizens. He is buried in Mount Wood Cemetery,

Wheeling, Ohio County, West Virginia. Thoburn distinguished himself as a surgeon and soldier who, like many other immigrants, gave his life to his adopted country.

Some soldiers who were wounded in the war and survived lived with disability or died later because of their injuries. One of these was a physician who lived with a disability and later died as a result of his battlefield injury. His name is **James Kiernan** (1837–1869) who was born in Mountbellew, County Galway to a retired surgeon in the British Navy. Kiernan attended Trinity College, Dublin, before emigrating to the US around 1854. At the outbreak of the Civil War, he joined the 69th New York Infantry Regiment as Assistant Surgeon and participated in the battle of the First Bull Run. During an interview with Lincoln, Kiernan made a promise to turn thousands of Irish-American Copperheads "into good union men." He served in the 6th Missouri Infantry Regiment at Pea Ridge, Arkansas. Kiernan insisted on joining the fighting ranks and was appointed a Major in the 6th Missouri. In 1863, at the Battle of Port Gibson Mississippi (April –May), he was shot in in the left shoulder and chest; the second bullet pierced his lung. He was left for dead on the field in a swamp. On recovery, he was captured by Confederate troops and imprisoned but escaped **(Fig 14)**. He resigned his commission, but in 1863, was re-commissioned as brigadier general of Volunteers by President Lincoln and charged with a post at Milliken's Bend on the Mississippi. Sickness from his battlefield wounds forced him to again resign in 1864. In 1865, he accepted a US consular post at Chinkiang in China. His continued ill-health compelled him to return to New York, where he became an examining physician for the Pension Bureau and continued serving in that capacity until his death.

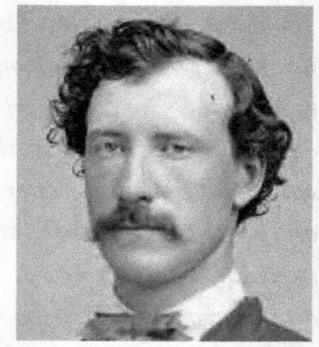

Fig 14. Irish-immigrant surgeon James Kiernan during the Battle of Port Gibson, Mississippi, survived after shots in the left shoulder and chest but died later from his war injury. (Find a Grave)

The reported cause of death was "congestion of the lungs" due to war wounds. He is buried in Green-Wood Cemetery in Brooklyn, New York.

Two other young Irish-American surgeons joined the Union Army and served with great courage exposing themselves to enemy fire in the midst of the battlefield, one of them was awarded the Medal of Honor.

Richard Curran (1838–1915) was born in the town of Ennis, County Clare, and emigrated with his parents to the US in 1850. He attended Harvard Medical School, graduating in 1859. At the beginning of the war, he raised two volunteer companies (A and K) from Seneca Falls, New York, and joined the 33rd New York Infantry in 1861, becoming an assistant surgeon in 1862. He was awarded the Medal of Honor for courage during the Battle of Antietam, where he was the regiment's only medical officer present on the battlefield. When the 33rd New York Infantry was disbanded in 1863, he continued service by joining the 6th New York Cavalry and later became the regimental surgeon of the 9th New York Cavalry, serving until the surrender of Robert E. Lee at Appomattox Court House. Curran participated in several other battles, including Fredericksburg and Chancellorsville, along with the Seven Day Battles. He voluntarily exposed himself to great danger by going to the frontlines to rescue wounded soldiers in the line of fire and directing them to the field hospital. Following the war, Curran opened a drugstore in Rochester, New York where he also participated in local Republican Party politics, winning the election to the New York State Assembly in 1891. He subsequently became Mayor of Rochester in 1892, serving a two-year term. He was buried in Holy Sepulchre Cemetery in Rochester.

William Blackwood (1838–1922) was born in Hollywood, County Wicklow, and emigrated to the US to study medicine at the University of Pennsylvania Medical School in 1859, graduating in 1862. In the same year, he enlisted into the 149th Pennsylvania Volunteer Infantry as Assistant Surgeon but was later transferred to the 48th Pennsylvania Infantry in 1863 as Chief Surgeon. During the deadly Third Battle of Petersburg when Fort Mahone was attacked on April 2, 1865, the regiment lost several men including its commander, and many were wounded. During the heat of the battle, Blackwood raced to the frontlines to assist seriously wounded officers and soldiers. He removed severely injured soldiers from the field while under heavy enemy fire, exposing himself beyond the call of duty, and demonstrating extraordinary gallantry. He also saw the war through to its conclusion. Following the war, Blackwood remained active in veterans' affairs, especially the 48th Veteran Association. He delivered the address at the regiment's monument at Antietam in 1904. Blackwood was subsequently awarded the Medal of Honor for his heroism. He died in Philadelphia and his remains are interred at the Chelten Hills Cemetery, Philadelphia.

English-Born Immigrant Physicians

We know of at least six English-born physicians who answered the call of duty and served during the war. We have limited information about three of them who served in the Union Army: **Robert Addison** (1803-1876), **Alfred Baker** (1813-1895) and **Edward Kittoe** (1814-1887).

One English-born artist and fearless physician who fought in the Civil War was recognized as the first Union medical officer killed in action. He is **Samuel Everett** (1820–1862) who first came to Quincy in 1840 with his family. He received medical training in St Louis. After a period of practice, he enlisted in 1861, as the regimental surgeon for the 10th Illinois Infantry. He reported to Cairo, where he was promoted to brigade surgeon of the 2nd Division. He then became medical director of the 2nd Division of the Army of the West and was assigned to duty at the US Army's 4th Street General Hospital in St. Louis. In 1862, he left St Louis and reported for duty at the headquarters of the Army of Tennessee, located three miles from Pittsburg Landing. He was assigned to the position of Brigade Surgeon for the 6th Division.

On Sunday morning, April 6, 1862, Everett was killed in the Battle of Shiloh in Hardin County, Tennessee while gallantly cheering on his men and encouraging them to renew their efforts to repulse the overwhelming waves of rebels attacking their division. He was hit by musket balls in the head and in the body. His horse was found shot dead about half a mile away. He is buried in Woodland Cemetery, Quincy, Adams County, Illinois.

Everett fearlessly exposed his life to enemy fire on the battlefield to save the wounded and proved his devotion to his country's cause by sacrificing his life on the battlefield. Besides having a reputation for being an eminent surgeon, he was also a talented artist and left behind him a litany of fabulous drawings, from his teenage years through the war years. Some of his works include: "*Camp at Lamine River, near Otterville,*" "*Fort Prentiss. Cairo*" and "*Military Ball.*" He was also a gifted writer and storyteller as is attested in many of the letters he wrote to family and friends.

One physician who was active in the Civil War is best known for helping to establish the practice of homeopathy in the Americas. Homeopathy is a controversial alternative treatment where practitioners use diluted substances that cause symptoms of a disease in healthy people and administer it to sick people with similar symptoms. Homeopaths believe this cures disease. This doctrine originated in Germany in the 18th century. The first homeopathic school in the US opened in 1835 and the American Institute of Homeopathy was established in 1844. Today, there is a lack of convincing scientific evidence to support the efficacy of homeopathic remedies. **Samuel Jones** (1834–1912) was originally born in Manchester, England and emigrated with his parents to America in 1842. He graduated in 1860 from the Missouri Homeopathic Medical College, St Louis, and subsequently from the Homeopathic Medical College of Pennsylvania, a year later. He practiced his profession during the war, when he served in the Union Army as First Assistant Surgeon of the 22nd New Jersey Infantry

(1862–63), and later as Assistant Surgeon of the 22nd Regiment of the New York State National Guard.

After the War, he became a professor at the New York Homeopathic Medical College, and later served as Dean at University of Michigan. Jones not only had a passion for homeopathy and teaching, but also a fascination with literature and book collecting, mainly from 19th century literary works. He kept extensive collections of English and American authors. He died in Ann Arbor, Michigan and is buried in Forest Hill Cemetery, Ann Arbor.

Most immigrant physicians during the Civil War were against slavery. One was a prominent abolitionist who also introduced a method of artificial respiration that helped save many soldiers and became widely used in the US. **Benjamin Howard** (1836–1900) was born in Chesham, England. After his parents passed, he was raised in another couple's household. On finishing school, he earned a living as a painter and wallpaper hanger. In 1853, he emigrated to America and attended Williams College in Massachusetts with the intention of becoming a medical missionary. He moved to New York and enrolled in Columbia University and received his degree in medicine in 1858.

After reading *Uncle Tom's Cabin* in the early 1850s, he secured a job as a clerk in a slave market in St Louis, Missouri, where he witnessed the horrors of the slave trade firsthand. He worked undercover for the Underground Railroad, helping slaves escape to Canada. When the Civil War erupted, Howard volunteered as Assistant Surgeon in the 19th Regiment of New York Volunteers and later as Assistant Surgeon in the regular army, serving on the staff of Major General George McClellan. In 1862, the Union and Confederate armies clashed on South Mountain and then on the banks of Antietam Creek. Howard found himself working under the direction of Major Jonathan Letterman. During the Battle of Antietam, Howard provided valuable aid to Letterman, riding over the fields and reporting on the conditions of the Medical Department. During this battle, Howard and

Letterman treated injured soldiers at the Pry House and cared for mortally wounded high-ranking officers.

Following the Battle of Antietam, Howard served as a medical purveyor and was appointed acting medical director for the Department of Ohio, where he recommended a new mode of treatment for wounds of the chest and abdomen by sealing them and allowing the collapsed lung to expand. In 1864, Howard developed a field ambulance with additional rollers and semi-elliptical springs for a smoother ride, as well as adjustable internal springs and cushioned seats.

After the war, Howard moved to New York where he practiced medicine and surgery, publishing an essay entitled *The Direct Method of Artificial Respiration, or the Treatment of Persons Apparently Dead from Suffocation by Drowning or from Other Cause* (1871). It became known as Howard's Direct Method of Artificial Respiration and was adopted throughout the US. Around 1873, Howard returned to England and helped establish the London Ambulance Service, which was modeled on his prototype. For ten years, Howard studied prison systems around the world; and in 1888, he traveled extensively around prisons in the US, England, Germany, Russia, and Siberia. He wrote two books on the subject, *Life with Trans-Siberian Savages* (1893) and *Prisoners of Russia: A Personal Study of Convict Life in Sakhalin and Siberia* (1902). Howard returned to New York in poor health and died of liver disease. He is buried in Elberton, New Jersey.

Immigrant Physicians of Other Nationalities

We know little about some of them but they are worth mentioning; all served in the Union Army. **James Bryan** (1810-1881) from Wales, **Eugène Abadie** (1810–1874) from France and Navy surgeon **William L Harkness** (1837-1903) of Scotland (Chapter 6), not to be confused with **William H Harkness** a non-physician immigrant killed in the war.

Two immigrant Norwegian relatives, anti-slavery advocates, one of them shot dying in action while the other a physician tried unsuccessfully to save his life. They are **Hans Christian Heg** (1829–1863) and **Stephen Himoe** (1832–1904). **Heg** was born in Haugestad, and while a child, he moved with his family to America in 1840, residing in the Muskego Settlement in Wisconsin. Heg became an outspoken anti-slavery activist and a leader of Wisconsin's Wide Awakes, an anti-slave catcher militia. In 1859, he was elected commissioner to the state prison in Waupun and became the first Norwegian-born candidate elected statewide in Wisconsin. Heg **(Fig 15)** spearheaded many reforms to the prison. In 1860, at great risk to his career, he provided shelter to Sherman Booth, a federal fugitive who had incited a mob to rescue an escaped slave.

With the outbreak of the Civil War, Heg was appointed by the Wisconsin Governor as Colonel of the 15th Wisconsin Infantry Regiment. Appealing to his fellow Norsemen, he said, *"The government of our adopted country is in danger. It is our duty as brave and intelligent citizens to extend our hands in defense of the cause of our Country and of*

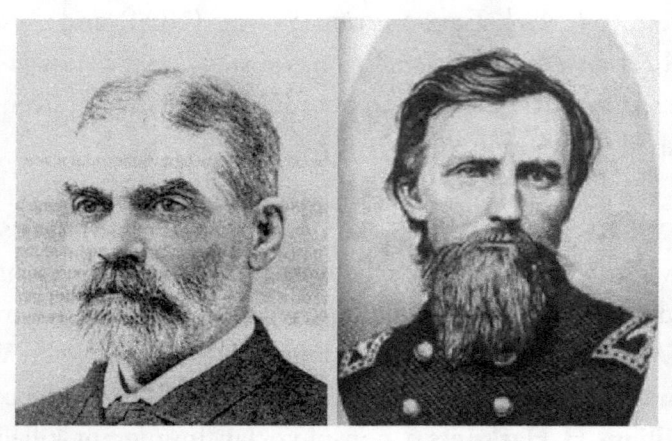

Fig 15. Scandinavian Regiment Surgeon Stephen Himoe (left) tended to his brother-in-law Norwegian-immigrant Hans Heg (right) as he lay dying from abdomen gunshot wound after the Battle of Chickamauga. (Wikipedia)

our homes." The company became known as the Scandinavian Regiment and the only of its kind because its soldiers were almost all immigrants from Norway, with some from Denmark and Sweden. Colonel Heg led his regiment into its first action at the Battle of Perryville. Despite being under fire from the enemy, the regiment suffered few casualties and no fatalities, but Heg was injured when his horse fell. Heg also saw action during the Battle of Stones River and in the Tullahoma campaign of 1863.

On September 19, 1863, while Heg was leading his brigade at the Battle of Chickamauga, he was struck in the abdomen by a Confederate sharpshooter's rifle. He rallied his troops but eventually had to relinquish his command. He was taken to a field hospital at Crawfish Spring, where he died on the second day. One of his attending surgeons who witnessed the passing of Heg was his brother-in-law, **Stephen Himoe**.

Heg was one of five Wisconsinite colonels killed during combat in the Civil War. As Acting Brigadier General of the Third Brigade, he was the highest-ranking officer from Wisconsin killed in the Civil War. He is buried at the Norway Lutheran Church Cemetery near Wind Lake, Wisconsin.

A statue of Hans Christian Heg was installed in 1925 near the State Capitol in Madison. Despite Heg being a staunch anti-slavery man, rioters from Black Lives Matter shamefully pulled his statue down, vandalized, decapitated, and threw it into Lake Monona. The unsalvageable statue was later recovered by the authorities. In 2020, the Wisconsin Capitol and Executive Residence Board voted unanimously to restore Heg's statue by creating a new one modeled on the statue of Heg in the town of Norway. In 2021, the Statue was reinstated.

Himoe moved from the Kingdom of Norway to the US in 1856 and graduated from St Louis Medical College. He settled in Kansas and practiced medicine in Lawrence, Douglas County. At the beginning of war, he served as military Surgeon in the 6th Kansas Cavalry and was appointed by the Wisconsin Governor as Surgeon to the

15th Wisconsin Volunteer Infantry, also known as The Scandinavian Regiment. Himoe **(Fig 15)**, was also reportedly Surgeon in the 24th Regiment of Kansas State Militia at Fort Scott. He was mustered into Federal service at Camp Randall near the City of Madison, Wisconsin. As the regiment's Surgeon, Himoe had a small medical staff but helped in caring for the injured. Himoe participated in the successful siege of Island 10 on the Mississippi River in Tennessee and the surprise raid on Union City, Tennessee in 1862. He also participated in the grueling 400-mile retreat to Louisville, Kentucky; the last two weeks of this retreat, they were on half rations and short of water. He also tended to his brother-in-law, **Colonel Heg**, as he lay dying from his wounds in the 1st Division Field Hospital at Crawfish Springs, Georgia, after the Battle of Chickamauga.

In late 1863, Himoe joined the 1st Division Hospital in Chattanooga which he later consolidated into a General Hospital. In the same year, the Army Medical Examining Board in Ohio summoned him to become Surgeon of Volunteers. The regiment's only remaining doctor died, leaving Himoe as the sole surgeon. Himoe resigned from the Army and returned to his family, moving to Fort Scott, Kansas, where he resumed his private medical practice for the remainder of his life.

Himoe was antislavery and one of his great nonmilitary accomplishments was in 1857, when he and five men organized a new company to lay out the town of Eldora—later called Mapleton, where he was appointed the first postmaster. He died of pneumonia and his body rests at the Oak Hill Cemetery in Lawrence, Douglas County Kansas.

One immigrant surgeon dedicated most of his career to educating the blind and introducing the Braille system to his students; he was also a champion of female doctors in his state. His name was **Simon Pollak** (1814–1903) and he was born in Prague, Bohemia. His family moved to Vienna where he graduated from medical school in 1835. He received postgraduate training in several different European cities. Pollak moved to the US in 1838 and practiced medicine in Nashville,

Tennessee, for several years. Pollak then accompanied Colonel Zachary Taylor, the future US president, on a trip to Louisiana, where he introduced him to influential people. Based on these contacts, Pollak moved to St Louis in 1844 and established a successful medical practice. He was a general practitioner but had a special interest in eye and ear diseases and is described as the first ophthalmologist in St Louis. Pollak served several terms as treasurer of the St Louis Medical Society and one term as its president.

At this time, the state of Missouri issued no funds for the education of the blind, and the state legislature took the stance that it was wasteful to educate the blind. By 1851, a private citizen, Eli Whelan, collaborated with Pollak to start a foundation called the Missouri School for the Blind. The organization applied for state funding, and the legislature later agreed to provide partial funding. The Missouri School for the Blind opened in 1851. Pollak introduced Braille to his students, a system that was not fully embraced in the US until the early 1890s. In 1860, he opened the first eye and ear clinic in St Louis, which was based at Mullanphy Hospital.

During the war, Pollak worked with other doctors to create the Western Sanitary Commission, which brought sanitary conditions to hospitals and trained nurses in military camps. The organization founded a total of fifteen hospitals in St Louis. Dr Pollak also championed the role of female doctors in the St Louis medical community. He served on the US Sanitary Commission, a private relief agency created by federal legislation in 1861, to support sick and wounded soldiers and volunteers of the US Army during the war. In 1863, he was appointed general hospital inspector of the US Sanitary Commission. After the war, he worked at the eye and ear clinic until his death, by which time he was considered the first ophthalmologist in St Louis and the most prominent member of the St Louis Medical Society.

Our next profile will be of a surgeon who served in the war, worked as a missionary, and even converted a steamer into a hospital ship to provide free healthcare for the poor and for drug addicts. Most importantly, he waged a relentless war against drug dealers and prompted his City Council to pass ordinances against selling opiates without a prescription. His name is **Alexander De Soto** (1840–1936) and he was born in the Caroline Islands, a Spanish colony at the time. His father was a general in the Spanish military, Spanish minister of war, and governor of the Caroline Islands. Alexander was also a great-great-grandson of Hernando de Soto, the Spanish explorer who first discovered the Mississippi River. He received a Doctor of Medicine degree from the University of Madrid in Spain and engaged in further studies in Heidelberg, Germany and Uppsala, Sweden. In 1862, De Soto came to the US and served as a navy surgeon during the war, working in Alaska. After the war, he travelled to Europe and practiced medicine but became addicted to gambling. In 1880, he returned to the US, moving between different cities and eventually quit gambling and engaged in missionary work in New York City and Seattle. Investing his own money, he established The Wayside Mission Hospital in 1899, as the first free hospital in Seattle, which sheltered the poor, sick, addicts and the suicidal **(Fig 16)**. In 1901, the hospital served 50,000 meals—mostly free and partly subsidized by De Soto. In 1900, he and his society members expanded the missionary hospital and converted the steamer

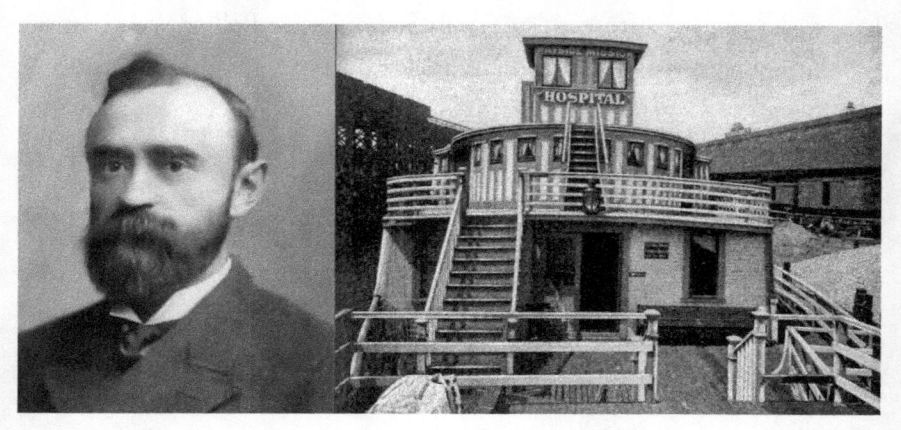

Fig 16. Spanish-American navy surgeon and missionary Alexander De Soto converted a steamer into the Wayside Hospital treating and sheltering for free the poor, sick, and addicts. (Wikipedia)

Idaho into a hospital ship, which offered space to treat 50 patients at a time and functioned as a rehabilitation center.

De Soto asked authorities to treat the city's drug addicts, and subsequently, ordinances were prepared that gave De Soto the authority to prevent the selling of any addictive drug without prescription. His relentless war against drug dealers prompted City Council to pass other ordinances that made selling opiates without a prescription a criminal offense. He convinced the city to keep drug addicts out of jails and instead admit them to his rehabilitation hospital. At first, the city council did not provide any funds for these programs; but later, a partnership was established between the City Council and De Soto's ship, which was named the *Wayside Emergency Hospital*. Again, because of the demand in 1903, he invested his own money in a four-story, brick-and-stone hospital. This was opposed by the county medical society and eventually he was ousted from his position and the ship hospital removed.

Later in his life, De Soto engaged in the mining and transportation business. He died after a fall and is buried in Seattle. De Soto the philanthropist is credited with building the Wayside Mission Hospital, the first public hospital in Seattle's history, which demonstrated the need for public health institutions and prompted the development of medical care for the homeless. In the 1920s, a historical plaque and an anchor marker were installed on the Washington Street Public Boat Landing in Seattle commemorating De Soto and the Wayside Mission Hospital.

The astounding story of the next immigrant surgeon is stranger than fiction. He was severely insane and yet profoundly erudite, making a unique contribution to the medical community through one of the greatest books ever published in the history of the English language. **William Chester Minor** (1834–1920) practiced medicine as an army surgeon in the war and saw action but did not himself fight. His insanity resulted from the horrors he witnessed on the battlefield, which after the war led him to commit a murder. While confined to a lunatic asylum, he became one of the most treasured lexicographers the English language has ever seen.

Minor had been born in Ceylon (Sri Lanka), the son of church missionaries. At the age of 14, he was sent to the US and lived with relatives in New Haven. He attended Russell Military Academy and subsequently enrolled at the Yale School of Medicine. While a medical student, he worked on the Webster's Dictionary. In 1863, he earned a medical degree with an emphasis on comparative anatomy. After a brief time at Knight General Hospital in New Haven, he had then joined the Union Army as a surgeon. Minor's grim task during the war was to try his best to save the lives of badly wounded soldiers by amputating limbs and digging out bullets, sometimes without anesthesia.

Deserters during the war were branded, tattooed, or even executed. In 1864, Lincoln spoke out against the execution of deserters, arguing that it was very difficult to shoot his own men. There are accounts placing Minor at the Battle of the Wilderness in 1864, which was notorious for the terrible casualties suffered by both sides. There is a story that Minor was given the task of punishing deserters by branding them with the letter D, including one Irish soldier, and that this latter incident played a role in his subsequent delusions.

After the war, Minor worked in New York City but began to show eccentric behavior including a fascination with the red-light district and its prostitutes. By 1868, his mental condition had deteriorated, and he was admitted to St Elizabeth Hospital, a lunatic asylum in Washington, DC. After 18 months without improvement, in 1871, Minor went to London to cure his mental condition, but he descended into an even worse madness and barricaded himself in a room. In 1872, haunted by his paranoia, he fatally shot George Merrett who had been on his way to work to support his six children and pregnant wife. Accounts vary as to why he shot Merrett; one suggests he thought him to be the Irish soldier he had branded and another that Minor wrongly believed Merrett was trying to break into his room.

After a trial, Minor (**Fig 17**) was found not guilty by reason of insanity and committed to the notorious asylum in Broadmoor, though he was given pleasant quarters and was allowed to read books. Minor heard a call for volunteers to contribute to writing for the *Oxford English Dictionary* (OED) and devoted the remaining two decades of his life to contributing to the publication, becoming one of the project's most important volunteers, compiling extensive quotations of words. Merrett's widow frequently visited him and even provided him with further books. Remorseful for the killing, he gave the widow most of his army pension. In 1899, James Murray the OED editor paid tribute to Minor's enormous contributions to the dictionary, stating, "We could easily illustrate the last four centuries from his quotations alone."

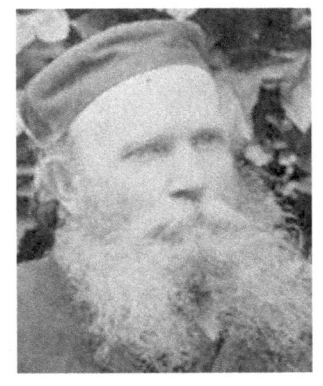

Fig 17. Ceylon-born immigrant erudite surgeon William Minor who became insane after the war and a key contributor to the Oxford English Dictionary. (Wikipedia)

Minor's condition continued to deteriorate, however. In 1902, while imagining he was sexually assaulting children, he used a knife to cut off his own penis to prevent this ever becoming a possibility. Murray campaigned on Minor's behalf and secured his release in 1910 on the orders of a then 35-year-old Winston Churchill. Minor returned to the US and resided at St Elizabeth Hospital, where he was diagnosed with schizophrenia. He died in a retreat for elderly persons with mental health disorders in Hartford, Connecticut, and was buried in Evergreen Cemetery in New Haven, Connecticut. Doctor Minor's story is depicted in a movie "The Professor and the Mad Man".

Psychological trauma of war is known to affect soldiers in what is known as post-traumatic stress disorder, but medical professionals serving in conflicts, encountering and caring for horrific war injuries are not immune to such mental distress and burnout.

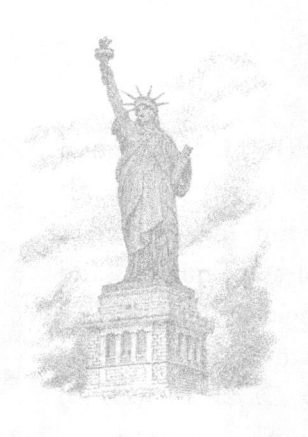

CHAPTER 6

Antebellum Physicians with Non-medical Contributions

Three immigrant physicians described earlier made noteworthy non-medical innovations worth mentioning here.

Ninety-three years before the New York State Legislature authorized construction of the Ere Canal in 1817 and over a century before its completion, an Irish immigrant physician asked to build a canal to connect the Hudson River with the Great Lakes to enhance fur trade with Native Americans and transport agricultural products to western settlers. This physician was **Cadwallader Colden** and as such he should be considered the seminal Father of the American Canal System. Colden was practicing medicine at the time in Philadelphia. After his canal proposal, he was invited by Robert Hunter, the colonial governor of New York, to relocate and become a surveyor general—a position he accepted in 1720. Colden became a politician and acting governor of New York. He published *An explication of the first causes of action in matter and of the cause of gravitation* (1745) in which he studied gravity, postulating a division of the material world into matter, light, and ether. He later wrote *Principles of Action in Matter, the gravitation of bodies, and the motion of the planets* (1751) and found fault with some of Isaac Newton's views.

One Irish immigrant surgeon **Thomas Antisell** also became renowned for his service to the Japanese Ministry of Finance and was commended for his developing of inks, in 1871, that could be used for printing paper currency. Antisell studied chemistry and geology, and after the war he became chief chemist in the US Department of Agriculture (1866–71), then Professor of Chemistry at Maryland Agricultural College (1869–70). Due to his background in chemistry and geology, Antisell was invited to join two other scientists on a US government commission whose task was to help develop the resources of Japan's northern islands. Because of a disagreement, he did not conclude his work, instead serving his time in the Empire of Japan as a chemist for the Ministry of Finance, where he developed inks for printing Japanese paper money. For his services, he was awarded the Order of the Rising Sun by Emperor Meiji before his return to the US in 1876, where he died in Washington DC.

Scottish-born immigrant Civil War physician Admiral **William Harkness** was appointed aide to the US Observatory, and later professor of mathematics. He became an accomplished astronomer and military scientist, serving as "aid in astronomy" at the US Naval Observatory (1862–65) and later the USS Monadnock (1865–66). During the total eclipse of the sun in 1869, he discovered the celestial sphere coronal line *K 1474*. His accomplishments include the construction of achromatic telescopes and invention of the spherometer caliper, along with other astronomical instruments. He designed enhanced photographic equipment and methods with improved accuracy for the measurement of distances between planets. His most celebrated non-medical publication is *The Solar Parallax and its Related Constants* (1891). Harkness died in Jersey City, New Jersey.

The following are stories of five other immigrant physicians who scarcely practice their medical profession, instead becoming best-known for their laudable contributions in nonmedical fields.

One immigrant British physician submitted an architectural design for the US Capitol in the City of Washington, competing with two world-renowned architects. This physician, who never had formal architectural training and was a self-taught architect, won the competition and went on to design several other prominent buildings; his name was **William Thornton** (1759–1828). Thornton was born in the British Virgin Islands in a Quaker community and at the age of five was sent to England for education. He grew up among Quakers in northern Lancashire, where he received medical training through an apprenticeship (1777–81) to a physician and apothecary. This was followed by enrollment in a medical course at the University of Edinburgh in 1781, but he instead received his medical degree in 1784 from the University of Aberdeen, Scotland; a practice that was customary when a student studied at several medical centers before graduating from one.

At an early age and while still a medical student, Thornton exhibited an interest in fine arts and kept a journal. Besides his notes on medical treatments, he also made drawings and sketches of flora and fauna, portraits, landscapes, historical scenes, and machinery.

When Thornton, the heir to a sugar plantation, returned to his boyhood town and came face-to-face with the source of his family's income, he was troubled by the institution of slavery. Fueled by an anti-slavery sentiment, he emigrated to the US, first living in Philadelphia and later settling in Washington DC. Philadelphia's Quaker establishment and future president James Madison, who lodged with Thornton, looked favorably upon his efforts to speak out against slavery in Europe prior to his emigration. In 1788, Thornton became an American citizen.

In Washington DC, after a brief period of medical practice, Thornton reverted to his drawing and submitted a design to the architectural competition for the Library Company of Philadelphia's new hall, which he won. In 1792, Thornton learned of the design competitions for the US Capitol and the President's House that was to be erected on the banks of the Potomac River. Inspired by the east front of the Louvre in France and the Pantheon in Rome, Thornton submitted a design for the Capital building. Rather than a simple congress hall, George Washington and Thomas Jefferson wanted the Capitol to be a national temple. The administration examined the designs submitted by Thornton and two other renowned immigrant architects; eventually Thornton won the competition and received a prize of $500. Thornton was appointed by Washington as one of the three commissioners in charge of overseeing the construction of the first government building, including the Capitol. Despite minor changes and additions by two other architects, much of the final design of the façade of the Capitol remained Thornton's.

Thornton went on to design other buildings that were added to the National Register of Historic Places. The Octagon House of Colonel John Taylor III in Washington DC served as a temporary executive mansion after the 1814 burning of the White House by the British; it was also where President Madison signed the Treaty of Ghent, ending the War of 1812. Thornton designed the Woodlawn Mansion for Major Lawrence Lewis, a historic building in Mount Vernon, as well as Tudor Place for Thomas Peter. Thornton was summoned to Mount Vernon in December 1799, to treat an ailing George Washington, but he was unable to save him as he arrived after Washington's death. Thornton himself died and was buried in Congressional Cemetery in eastern Washington, DC.

The Scottish-born physician **James Tytler** (1745–1804) was plagued with repeated business failures that eventually led to his demise. The only success he had in life was at being a writer and lexicographer. He established a hot air balloon business, which failed, but it brought him fame for being the first man to fly a balloon in Britain. Tytler studied medicine at the University of Edinburgh and became apprenticed to a surgeon on a whaling ship for one year before deciding to pursue another career. He was not awarded a medical degree but practiced medicine briefly, before opening a pharmacy business that failed, forcing him into bankruptcy. To escape creditors, he left Scotland for England and worked under a pseudonym as an apothecary—a business that also failed. He prospered, however, as editor of the Encyclopedia Britannica for its second and third editions. His success was nevertheless ephemeral as he went bankrupt again, after engaging in the hot air balloon business. After a failed first attempt, he floated in a 40-foot tall, barrel-shaped balloon and became the first person in Britain to do that in 1784. On his third attempt, he crashed in front of hundreds of paying spectators—which also got him into financial trouble.

Tytler emigrated in 1795 to the US after being outlawed in absentia for sedition by the Scottish High Court for his liberal views. In Salem, Massachusetts, he edited the *Salem Register* and published a newspaper called *Universal Geography*, an ancestor of the *National Geographic*. Tytler was an avid reader and prolific author of many anonymous works and popular songs. His contributions to medicine include a publication on the *System of Surgery* and *A treatise on the plague and yellow fever* (1799). Tytler came to a bad end, slipping into the sea when drunk and drowning near Salem, Massachusetts. It took two days for the sea to return his body to shore.

The history of the ice making mechanism began with Oliver Evans, the American inventor who described the concept of refrigeration in 1805 using a vapor-compression machine. In 1834, Jacob Perkins built the first refrigerating machine, which used ether in a vapor compression cycle. However, it was an immigrant physician who first built a refrigerator based on Oliver Evans' original concept and produced ice. His invention was initially intended to cool the air for his yellow fever patients. His idea dates to 1842, making him one of the founding fathers of the refrigerator.

IMMIGRANT PHYSICIANS

John Gorrie (1803–1855) was born in the same birthplace as Alexander Hamilton on the Island of Nevis in the West Indies to Scottish parents. He moved with his family during childhood to South Carolina where he then grew up. He received his medical degree in 1827 from the College of Physicians and Surgeons in Fairfield, New York. In 1833, he moved to Florida, where he worked as resident physician at two hospitals. He became active in his community in a dizzying array of roles, serving as a council member, postmaster, bank president, secretary of a masonic lodge, and became one of the founders of the Trinity Episcopal Church.

Gorrie (**Fig 18**) also conducted research on tropical diseases, particularly malaria and yellow fever. To control the disease and the fever, Gorrie urged draining the swamps following beliefs of the time regarding its origin. He also tried cooling patients' sickrooms with ice in a basin suspended from the ceiling. To do this, he began experimenting with making artificial ice. In 1844, he made the first mechanically produced ice. Gorrie then gave up his medical practice to pursue his new refrigeration enterprise. By 1850, he was able to routinely produce ice the size of bricks. In 1851, he was granted a patent for an ice-making machine. However, in 1835, a patent for "Apparatus and means for

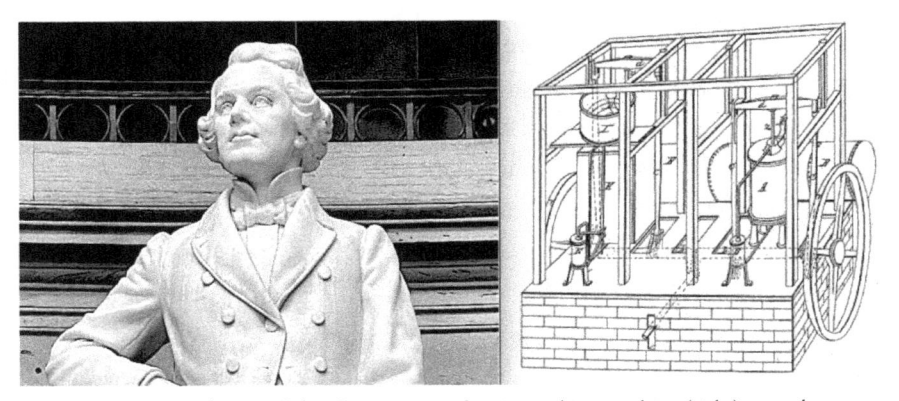

Fig 18. Immigrant physician John Gorrie patented an ice-making machine (right) to cool rooms of febrile patients, which was the precursor to the air-conditioning and refrigeration systems. (Public domain)

producing ice and in cooling fluids" had been granted in Europe to American-born inventor Jacob Perkins. Gorrie had the right idea, but he was unable to capitalize on it. Unfortunately, his plans for manufacturing and selling ice were also met with fierce opposition from Frederic Tudor, the Boston "Ice King." Gorrie also failed to raise money to manufacture his machine. He became impoverished and then financially ruined, his health deteriorated, and he died and was buried in Magnolia Cemetery.

A version of Gorrie's "cooling system" was used when President James Garfield was dying in 1881 from an infected bullet wound. To lower his fever, naval engineers built a large box filled with cloths that had been soaked in melted ice water. Blowing air onto the cloths decreased the overall room temperature. The problem with this method was what Gorrie had encountered; it required a large amount of ice to keep the room cooled continuously. Gorrie's invention nevertheless was an important event in the history of air conditioning. The first practical refrigeration system was patented four years after Gorrie's patent and built by James Harrison in Australia (1855).

Gorrie did not receive the recognition he deserved while alive, but he did earn several formal acknowledgments of his work posthumously. In Apalachicola, Florida, Gorrie Square is named in his honor and contains his gravesite. A monument, a state museum, a municipal library, and a bridge across Apalachicola Bay were all named after him. In 1914, the state of Florida also gave a statue of Gorrie to the National Statuary Hall Collection. Other eponyms he earned include a High School in Jacksonville, an elementary school in Tampa, and even the ship SS John Gorrie. Finally, the John Gorrie Award is given each year to a graduate of the University of Florida College of Medicine.

Below are two final stories of immigrant surgeons who made significant new inventions.

The 'empty sleeve' became a metaphor for veterans who lost hands and then returned to 'normal' life after the Civil War. Among their many challenges were basic daily activities like eating with a knife and fork—which requires two hands. One surgeon thought that one of the most useful tools for an upper-limb amputee would be an eating utensil used in one hand. He therefore designed a device based on a utensil belonging to Admiral Horatio Nelson of the British Royal Navy after he lost his arm in 1797. The knife became an essential tool for one-armed veterans to eat unassisted. The immigrant surgeon responsible was **William Detmold** (1808–1894) who was born in Hanover, Germany, receiving his medical degree from the University of Göttingen in 1830 and enlisting as surgeon in the royal Hanoverian grenadier-guard. In 1837, Detmold went to the US on a leave of absence and sent back his resignation from New York City where he remained for the rest of his life. In 1841, he established one of the earlier orthopedic clinics in New York. After serving in the Civil War, he became interested in amputation and rehabilitation technology for war veteran amputees. During the war, he introduced the knife-fork to one-armed amputee soldiers, and it became known as "Detmold's knife. The knife, used by the remaining hand, is steel with a wooden handle and included a soft case for carrying when dining outdoors. The Detmold knife was manufactured by a New York company and was supplied by the US Government to Civil War veterans. One of his other important medical contributions was to introduce orthopedic surgery to the US as a surgical specialty. His civil engineer immigrant brother **Christian** helped laying the foundations of Fort Sumter.

The military surgical career of **Simon Baruch** (1840–1921) was discussed earlier. After immigrating in 1855 to the US from Prussia, he graduated from the Medical College of Virginia, in Richmond. After serving on the Confederate side during the war and during the Reconstruction Era, he made Camden his home. He then became a medical writer, publishing about war injuries, specifically Bayonet Wounds. While practicing medicine, he also cared for the poor and thousands of arriving immigrants living in New York slums who lacked access to proper bathing facilities. Even a simple sponge bath was a luxury for residents in crowded apartments without bathrooms, who had to carry buckets of water to stoves. Unsurprisingly, morbidity and mortality rates were high among these residents. Baruch made it his mission for years to establish public bathhouses in New York City and introduced a novel form of treatment called hydrotherapy. He published three books on the topic and became a public health advocate in New York. In 1895, he successfully persuaded the State Legislature to pass a law requiring cities with a minimum population of 50,000 to establish and maintain free bathhouse facilities

In 1901, Baruch **(Fig 19)** and his colleagues presided over the opening of the first free public bathhouse, the Rivington Street Municipal Bath, in Manhattan. Other public baths were built and credited to Baruch's advocacy. Simon Baruch is the namesake of civil monuments, educational entities, and academic departments in New York City and around the country, including public housing complex in Manhattan, academic chairs at three universities. His name also graces the New York City Department of Education, a middle school and adjacent playground and garden. In 1933, the Simon Baruch Research Institute of Balneology at Saratoga Springs, New York was established. Baruch's

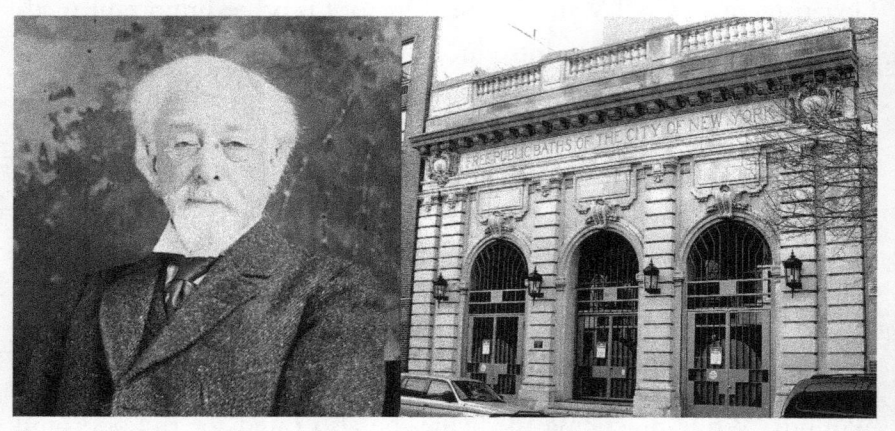

Fig 19. Simon Baruch German immigrant physician who cared for thousands of New York City poor and immigrants and built many free public bathhouses, one seen on the right. (Wikipedia)

name has been given to an auditorium on the campus of the Medical University of South Carolina in Charleston, the Department of Physical Medicine and Rehabilitation at Virginia Commonwealth University, and the Egyptian Building, now a National Historic Landmark.

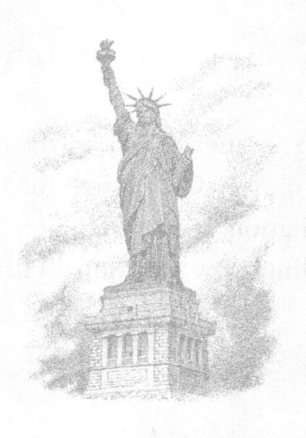

CHAPTER 7

Physicians at the Dawn of Modern Medicine

During the post-Civil War Reconstruction period in the mid-19th to 20th centuries, immigrants spread across America, bringing with them varied experiences and perspectives. They became loyal citizens who helped rebuild the country's systemic and scientific makeup. Among them were physicians or future physicians who made landmark contributions to advance medical science, bridging the way to modern American medicine with its global reach.

From Small Town Clinic to Global Medical Center

A boy was born in England and emigrated to the US, becoming a physician in Rochester, Minnesota. Due to his stature, he became known as the "little doctor." After a tornado hit the city and caused many injuries, this solo practitioner, with the help of an immigrant Roman Catholic nun, decided to start a clinic to assist the people of his small community. Today, this physician has become a giant in his field, and his clinic is renowned worldwide as a nonprofit American academic medical center for healthcare, education, and research. It has recently been ranked number one in the US for six consecutive years. **William Worrall Mayo** (1819–1911) was born in Eccles, Lancashire, the same year as the Peterloo Massacre took place in St. Peter's Square, Manchester, a time of economic and political upheaval. Mayo **(Fig 20)** left Britain for the US in 1846 and initially worked as a pharmacist at Bellevue Hospital in New York City. He began his medical career in 1849 by studying medicine at Indiana Medical College in La Porte and graduated in 1854 from the University of Missouri with a degree in medicine.

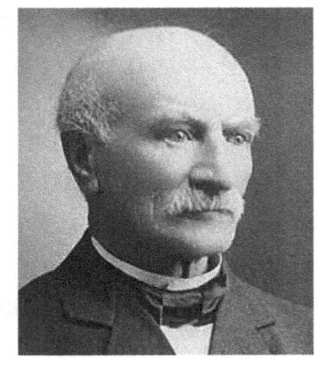

Fig 20. British–born William Worrall Mayo began as a solo practitioner in a small town; his big vision led him to build a vast clinic with reputation and reach across the world. (Wikipedia)

Mayo settled in Minnesota, and during the American Civil War, he was denied becoming an army surgeon. However, he managed to volunteer in a makeshift hospital caring for the war injured, and with his wife, they hosted refugees. While in solo practice, he continued studying in New York and Pennsylvania to improve his surgical skills by dissecting cadavers of executed men. Mayo had two sons, William and Charles, who also became physicians. During that time, he also immersed himself in politics and served as a city mayor and later as a Minnesota state senator. After a tornado devastated Minnesota, Mayo asked the Sisters of St. Francis to help, and along with his sons, they provided care to the disaster victims.

Mother Alfred Moses, a Luxembourg-born immigrant of the Sisters of St. Francis, believed that a hospital was needed in Rochester and asked Mayo to administer it. She raised the necessary funds to build the hospital and supervised its construction. Thanks to her vision, direction, and collaboration with Mayo, St. Mary's Hospital, originally with 12 beds, was built and began operations in 1889, with Mayo and his two sons as surgeons, and the Sisters of St. Francis as staff. Before his retirement, Mayo created the nucleus of the Mayo Clinic by inviting Augustus Stinchfield to join him in practice, which later grew into a group of physicians, including the Canadian-American **Donald Balfour** (1882–1963), who eventually became the Director of the Mayo Foundation for Medical Education and Research and married Mayo's daughter. The Mayo brothers were instrumental in establishing today's Mayo Clinic. Mayo suffered a crushing injury to his hand while conducting research, and his sons cared for his wound, which became infected and required amputation. This complication led to his death at nearly the age of 92. Today, Mayo Clinic is Dr. Mayo's legacy and as of 2022, it has over 63,000 employees, including 4,500 physicians and scientists, across three major campuses.

How Pediatrics Became a Specialism

The American Medical Association (AMA) is a professional medical organization and lobbying group for physicians, headquartered in Chicago, Illinois. With a membership exceeding 270,000 in 2021, it is one of the largest medical organizations in the world. Founded in 1847, the AMA's first president was Nathanial Chapman. From its inception until 2022, a total of 177 physicians have served as its presidents, all of whom were Americans with one known immigrant, **Abraham Jacobi** (1830-1919), who was born to Jewish parents in Hartum, Germany seventeen years before the AMA was founded. Jacobi studied medicine and graduated with a medical degree in 1851 from the University of Gottingen in Bonn. He was apprehended twice by the Prussian authorities for joining the German Revolution in 1848, and later he left for England where he stayed with Karl Marx and Friedrich Engels. He then emigrated to the US and arrived in New York City in 1853, where he practiced medicine with a focus on pediatrics. He remained in contact with Marx and Engels and helped found the New York Communist Club in 1857.

In 1855, Jacobi began lecturing on childhood diseases, and in 1860, he became the professor and chair of the first discipline in the US, infantile pathology, and therapeutics, at the New York Medical College. He thus created a new branch of medicine for the treatment of children's diseases, which became known as pediatrics. Jacobi **(Fig 21)** taught at Columbia University and later moved to Mount Sinai Hospital, where he became a professor and established the first Department of Pediatrics and children's clinic in the country in 1862. During his lifetime, most teaching hospitals established pediatric departments. He was a key figure in the movement to improve American child healthcare and welfare. He was an educator advocating for bedside teaching and made extensive contributions to the medical literature, helping to create the American Journal of Obstetrics. He also championed the care of women's diseases and midwifery, advocating for breastfeeding and birth control. Jacobi is regarded as the "Father of American Pediatrics," and a medical center in New York City was named after him.

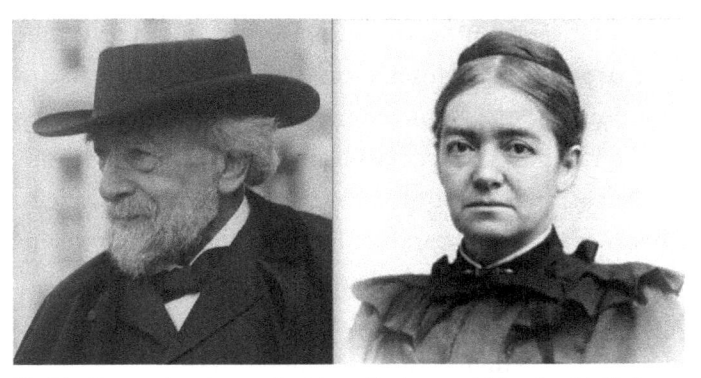

Fig 21. German immigrant physicians Abraham and Mary Jacobi. He is credited with establishing "Pediatrics" as a specialty in the US, she advocated for women's rights to medical education and both championed child and women's healthcare. (Wikipedia)

Jacobi was widowed twice, and his third wife was **Mary Jacobi (Fig 21)** (1842–1906), a British-born American who was the first woman to study medicine at the University of Paris. She was an esteemed American physician, teacher, scientist, writer, and suffragist who advocated for women's rights, particularly in medical education. She challenged the popular belief that menstruation made women unsuited for education, and she was a professor in the new Women's Medical College of the New York Infirmary and Mount Sinai Hospital, where she practiced medicine alongside her husband (Chapter 10).

From Coca Leaf to Pain Relief

Before the advent of anesthesia, surgery was a horrifying prospect for patients and grueling and prohibitive for surgeons. Surgeons relied on speed to perform amputations while restraining combative patients. The introduction of ether in 1846 and chloroform a year later offered patients the opportunity for humane and pain-free surgery. Today, anesthesia combines the use of intravenous drugs and inhaled gas, such as nitrous oxide, to render the patient in a state of deep unconsciousness during major operations.

The cornea or white portion of the human eye has profuse pain sensation emanating from nerve endings called nociceptive fibers. Even the presence of an eyelash causes a foreign body response in the eye that can be very bothersome. Some surgeries, including certain eye procedures, require the patients' cooperation while awake, without general anesthetic. Performing eye surgery while the patient is awake is difficult not only because of the discomfort but also the involuntary reflex that causes the eye to move in response to the slightest touch.

A Viennese ophthalmologist who emigrated to America discovered a method where a medicine can be applied locally to the eye to eliminate sensation and allow manipulating, injecting or even cutting the eye tissue, while the patient is awake without pain. His introduction of surface anesthetic in eye surgery in 1884 inaugurated the modern era of local anesthesia. This physician's name is **Karl Koller** (1857-1944), and he was born in Schüttenhofen, Bohemia. Koller began his medical career as a house surgeon at the Vienna General Hospital working with colleague Sigmund Freud. When Freud, attempted to cure a friend of morphine addiction, he asked Koller to investigate the physiological effects of cocaine as a possible remedy. The numbing effect of chewing coca leaves had long been recognized by Inca medicine men who sucked coca leaf along with vegetable ash and dripped saliva into the wounds of injured worriers for pain relief. Koller diverted his experimental research towards his specialty and used solutions such as chloral hydrate and morphine as anesthetics in the eyes of laboratory animals without success. He then used coca leaves and his results convinced him that cocaine has a numbing effect on the eye and it could be used as a local anesthetic in eye surgery.

Koller's findings were a medical breakthrough and a godsend not only to ophthalmologists but other surgeons as well. In the 20th century, agents such as lidocaine have replaced cocaine as a local anesthetic in many medical fields from dermal to dental surgery and from obstetric to orthopedic surgery. In 1888, prompted by anti-Semitism, Koller moved to the US and until the 1930s engaged in private practice as ophthalmologist at Mount Sinai and Montefiore Hospitals in New York where he married and settled permanently. In 1902, he became a citizen of the US. Koller authored many articles related to eye physiology and ophthalmology.

One of Koller's patients was a ten-year-old boy who was nearly blind named Chauncey Leake. Koller helped Leake recover his eyesight and as an adult Leake became a renowned American ethicist, medical historian and pharmacologist who went on to discover the anesthetic divinyl ether that has less adverse side effects and has quicker onset and recovery than ether; it continued to be used in some countries as a general anesthetic until the 1960s when it was found to have, with long-term use, liver and kidney toxicity. Nicknamed "Coca Koller" by Freud, Koller received many distinctions including gold medal from the American Ophthalmological Society, Medal of Honor from New York Academy of Medicine, Kussmaul Medal from Heidelberg University Germany, and the "Lucien Howe Medal" from the Medical Association of Vienna.

Controlling a Killer Epidemic

During the Spanish-American War of 1898, while the US Army was present in Cuba, an epidemic of yellow fever broke out in 1900 and infected 1,200 soldiers. The mode of transmission of the disease was unknown, with some believing it was of bacterial origin and others thinking it was contagious through touching dressings of an infected person. It wasn't until two immigrant Army physicians conducted research and found the cause of the disease to be a virus transmitted through mosquito bites. They also experimented with yellow fever vaccination, which eventually led to the control of the mosquito problem and the eradication of the disease from Cuba. Sadly, one of these physician scientists, **James Carroll** (1854-1907), died due to complications from yellow fever. Carroll, originally from England, had moved to Canada in 1874 and then to the US in the same year, enlisting in the Army to eventually become a General. He graduated with a medical degree in 1891 from the University of Maryland and studied bacteriology under William Welch at Johns Hopkins Hospital, assisting Army Physician Walter Reed in pathology laboratories. Carroll and Reed later worked together at the Army Medical Museum in Washington and the Columbia University Medical School.

In 1900, Carroll served as a member of the Yellow Fever Commission in Cuba, along with physicians Walter Reed, Jesse Lazear, and the immigrant-American **Aristides Agramonte**. During the experiments, Carroll and Lazear subjected themselves to mosquito bites loaded with yellow fever in order to prove that mosquitoes were disease carriers. Both physicians developed severe disease, with Lazear tragically dying, and Carroll recovering but suffering permanent heart complications as a result. Carroll's research proved that yellow fever is caused by a virus, not bacteria, making him the first to demonstrate that viruses can cause disease in humans. He also proved that blood from active cases of yellow fever contained the infective agents. The findings of the commission led to the control of the mosquito problem in Havana, and yellow fever was soon eradicated from Cuba.

Following his work on yellow fever, Carroll shifted his focus to studying typhoid fever, a bacterial infection, and developing a prophylactic vaccine. In 1904, with permission from Army Surgeon-General Robert O'Reilly, Carroll tested an oral typhoid fever vaccine on himself and 12 other military volunteers. Due to a faulty vaccine from laboratory preparation, seven men became ill, but all survived. However, the Office of the Surgeon General did not publicize the results. Although Carroll had recovered from his initial yellow fever infection, his heart was irreparably damaged, and he died seven years later. Despite the risks associated with the experiments on typhoid fever, they were conducted in an ethical manner by obtaining informed consent from the volunteers. Reed and Carroll thus began the tradition of ethical medical research in the US Army, aimed at protecting the health of the military.

Carroll's scientific research resulted in several books and articles that he wrote and co-authored, primarily on yellow fever. He was also the inaugural president of the US and Canadian Academy of Pathology. He was buried at Arlington National Cemetery in Arlington, Virginia. Overall, Carroll's contributions to medical research, particularly in the field of infectious diseases, left a lasting impact on the understanding and control of these diseases. He is remembered for his pioneering work in demonstrating the role of viruses in human diseases, as well as his ethical approach to medical research. His legacy continues to be recognized and honored in the field of pathology and beyond. Thanks to his efforts, many lives have been saved from deadly diseases. His work remains an important part of medical history. Rest in peace,

James Carroll. Your contributions to science and medicine will not be forgotten.

Building a trans-isthmian canal to efficiently transport goods between the Atlantic and Pacific coasts was a challenging goal for the US, Britain, and France. In 1850, negotiations with Britain for constructing an Anglo-American canal failed. French attempts to build a canal through Panama, which was part of Colombia at the time, made progress when Ferdinand de Lesseps, the builder of the Egyptian Suez Canal, began excavating in 1880. However, yellow fever and malaria plagued de Lesseps' campaign, and after nine years and the loss of about 20,000 lives, the French attempt was halted. It was President Theodore Roosevelt who eventually fulfilled the long-term US goal of building the canal, a project that began in 1903 and was completed in 1914. Before construction began, the yellow fever epidemic was in full swing, and during the early stages of construction, American builders of the canal faced similar challenges to those of the French. While erecting housing for thousands of railway workers, yellow fever, and malaria, transmitted by mosquitoes, took a toll, and 12,000 workers died. The construction of a railway to move supplies was halted due to the lack of healthy workers, which jeopardized the entire project.

In 1904, a Canal Commission headed by Colonel William Gorgas was created with the objective of ensuring the welfare of the workers by implementing a safety and sanitation program to combat disease. Four years earlier, a four-member Yellow Fever Commission led by Walter Reed was created in the US to study the transmission of the disease and control the Cuban epidemic. Dr. Gorgas capitalized on the findings of the Yellow Fever Commission from 1901, which were crucial for the success of the Canal Commission, and by 1906, yellow fever and malaria were virtually wiped out from the Canal Zone.

One of the members of the Yellow Fever Commission was the Cuban-American **Aristides Agramonte** (1868-1931), who was born the son of a prominent physician in an area now known as Camagüey. As a youngster, Agramonte moved with his family to New York, where he received early schooling and later graduated from the College of Physicians and Surgeons in 1892. After an internship at Roosevelt Hospital, he practiced at Bellevue Hospital and worked for the city health department. He specialized in pediatrics and worked in pathology and bacteriology laboratories, where he developed expertise in tropical medicine. Following the outbreak of the Spanish-American War, Agramonte enlisted in the US army as an acting assistant surgeon and was sent to Cuba in 1898 to study yellow fever, which caused death among soldiers. After the occupation of Havana, Agramonte took charge of the army medical laboratory.

The Yellow Fever Commission including Agramonte and Carroll **(Fig 22)** researched the yellow fever outbreak and its transmission in Cuba, where locals were more immune to the disease than American soldiers. The US government also intended to investigate and prevent acute infectious diseases including malaria that were occurring in Panama and might interfere with the construction of the Canal.

Reed returned to the US while the team conducted experiments on themselves, soldiers, and paid volunteers. As a result, Lazar died from yellow fever due to a self-inflicted mosquito bite. It was unclear whether Agramonte inoculated himself and did not contract the disease due to childhood immunity or if he simply did not expose himself to mosquito bites. However, his experience as a pathologist and bacteriologist, as well as his work during the Cuban yellow fever epidemic, greatly contributed to the success of the board by disproving the prevailing theory that a bacillus was the causative agent of yellow fever, and instead proving the earlier hypothesis of the Cuban epidemiologist Carlos Finlay that a virus was the culprit.

After completing the board's mission in 1901, Agramonte was discharged from the army and accepted a professorship of bacteriology and experimental pathology at the University of Habana. He

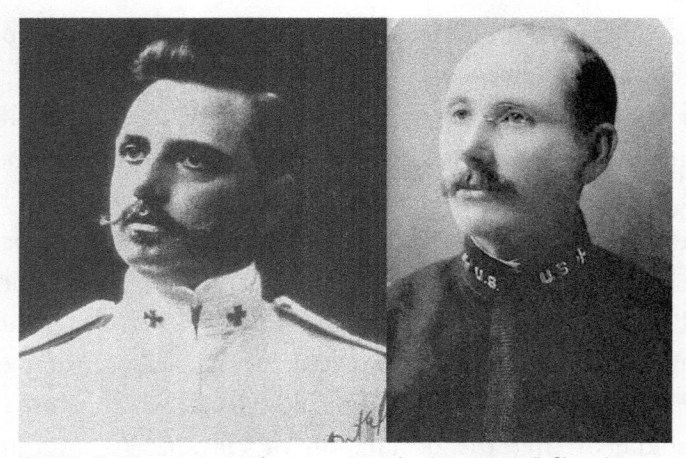

Fig 22. Immigrant Army physicians Aristides Agramonte (left) and James Carroll (right) members of the Yellow Fever Commission who found the mosquito as source and eradicated the disease from Cuba. (Wikipedia)

continued his studies on dengue, malaria, trachoma, typhoid fever, and other tropical diseases.

In 1931, the University of Louisiana medical school in New Orleans established a department of tropical medicine and invited Agramonte to head the department. He moved his family to New Orleans, where he worked until his death from a heart attack. Agramonte also served as the president of the Pan-American Medical Association and the president of the Columbia Alumni Club of Havana. In the 1920s, the U.S. Congress granted Aristides Agramonte the Merit of Honor medal and a monthly pension for his role in the yellow fever campaign.

Unraveling the Mysteries of Blood

Blood transfusion is a potentially life-saving procedure in which whole blood or its components are delivered to the circulation through a vein to replace blood lost from injury or surgery. It can also be used for certain blood diseases, such as iron deficiency anemia, sickle cell anemia, hemophilia, and thalassemia.

In the 17th century, attempts at blood transfusions from animal to animal were proven feasible, but transfusions in humans were problematic due to potentially life-threatening complications for the recipients. James Blundell, an English obstetrician, is credited with the first successful blood transfusion in 1829, from a husband to his heavily bleeding wife after childbirth. After conducting many transfusions, Blundell realized that some patients developed kidney failure and died. In 1881, William Halstead drew blood from his own arm and transfused it to his sister who was in hemorrhagic shock after giving birth, saving her life. Fortunately, she did not experience any complications from the procedure.

One major problem that physicians faced with blood transfusion was blood incompatibility or hemolytic transfusion reaction, which occurred when the recipient's antibodies attacked the transfused red blood cells. Earlier blood transfusions were often followed by shock and jaundice. However, this obstacle was overcome at the beginning of the 20th century when **Karl Landsteiner**, an Austrian-born American physician, made a discovery that allowed blood transfusion without the potential for hemolytic reaction. Landsteiner, who was born in Baden to Jewish parents but later converted to Roman Catholicism, grew up in Vienna and graduated from medical school in 1891 at the University of Vienna. He furthered his knowledge of chemistry and cancer antibodies by spending time in German and Swiss laboratories. In 1897, he became a professor at the University of Vienna, teaching anatomy and pathology and conducting thousands of cadaver dissections and autopsies. In 1908, along with the Austrian physician Erwin Popper, Landsteiner isolated the virus that causes poliomyelitis.

Landsteiner observed a pattern of antigen-antibody reaction that occurred when blood serum from different individuals was combined, causing red blood cells to burst. He continued his research to find the cause of this response and in 1901, he was the first to identify the three blood groups A, B, and O. He found that blood transfusion between patients with the same blood group did not cause destruction of blood cells, which made blood transfusion safe, marking a landmark breakthrough. However, another challenge was encountered.

In 1923, Landsteiner emigrated to the US and joined the Rockefeller Institute in New York. In 1929, he became a US citizen. While in New York, Landsteiner collaborated with his assistant, **Philip Levine**, an immune-hematologist who was a Russian-American physician. Together, they made another discovery in 1937. Levine published a case report in collaboration with another researcher about a mother who had a transfusion reaction and gave birth to a stillborn baby that died of hemolytic disease after receiving a blood transfusion from her husband during delivery, even though both parents had compatible blood group O. The conclusion was that there must be an undiscovered blood group antigen present in the husband's red blood cells but not in his wife's, which caused incompatibility between the mother's and fetus' blood.

In 1937, Landsteiner **(Fig 23)** learned that the cause of newborn death was the mother making a blood group antibody that sensitized her fetus' red blood cells. The term "Rh" was an abbreviation of "Rhesus factor," which Alexander Wiener believed at the time to be a similar antigen found in rhesus macaque monkey's red blood cells. The discovery of the Rh factor is the outcome of collaboration between more than one researcher, but Landsteiner's collaboration with Alexander Wiener led him to discover the factor.

Landsteiner's collaboration with Levine also refined his discovery by introducing new blood groups M, N, and P. Shortly thereafter, ABO blood groups began to be used for paternity testing to determine if an individual is the biological parent of another, which is important if the father's paternity of a child is in doubt. Today, DNA profiling is a more advanced technology for paternity testing. In 1943, Landsteiner had a heart attack while working in his laboratory and died two days later. In 1930, Landsteiner was awarded the Nobel Prize in Physiology or Medicine for his pioneering discovery of blood types. He became known as the "Father of Transfusion Medicine." He was posthumously inducted into the Polio Hall of Fame and awarded the Lasker-DeBakey Clinical Medical Research Award.

Jehovah's Witness religion is a Christian denomination with millions of followers worldwide. Although blood transfusion is a welcome lifesaving treatment for members of almost all religious groups, Jehovah's Witnesses prohibit their followers from having blood transfusions even in life-threatening situations because of their belief that it is against God's will. This has led to enormous challenges for the medical community when treating Jehovah's Witness patients, especially in children, where parents refuse transfusion knowing that it can make the difference between a child's life and death. A minority of Jehovah's Witnesses are open-minded about receiving blood substitutes or the reinfusion of their own blood. The refusal of blood transfusion has brought some cases to court hearings between hospitals and doctors versus Jehovah's Witness patients. In 1962, a New York state judge ruled in favor of a Jehovah's Witness patient against transfusion, and the patient died. In 1963, in another case, a Jehovah's Witness patient refused needed emergent transfusion for bleeding from a ruptured stomach ulcer, and the federal judge ruled in favor of the hospital, allowing the transfusion to be given. In 1965, the Illinois Supreme Court ruled in the case of the Estate of Brooks that the demanded transfusion for a Jehovah's Witness was an unconstitutional invasion of a person's religious beliefs.

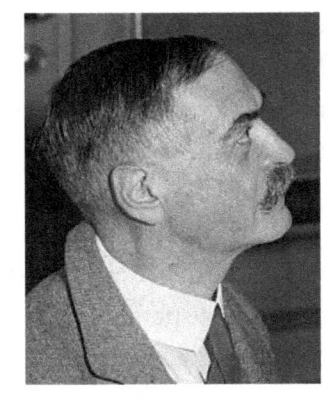

Fig 23. Immigrant anatomist and physician Karl Landsteiner "Father of Transfusion Medicine", identified ABO blood groups that made blood transfusion safely possible. He also discovered poliomyelitis virus. (Wikipedia)

Courts continue to struggle today, especially in the case of children facing life-threatening challenges, with whether to rule for or against transfusions. In the 1950s in Louisiana, it was illegal for physicians to transfuse a white patient with blood from a black person without prior permission.

Red blood cells are one of the components of blood, along with white cells, platelets, and plasma. Plasma is the liquid in which the cells are suspended. The cellular constituents of blood are formed in the bone marrow. White blood cells include granulocytes (neutrophils, eosinophils, and basophils), monocytes, and lymphocytes (T cells and B cells), and comprise the body's immune system, protecting it against infections and foreign invaders. All white blood cells are produced and derived from "multipotent" cells in the bone marrow known as hematopoietic stem cells. Platelets (thrombocytes), like red blood cells, do not have nuclei but are smaller; they are formed from megakaryocytes that reside in the bone marrow. Megakaryocytes are formed in the hematopoietic stem cell system. The process of hematopoiesis, which gives rise to other blood cells from stem cells, is of paramount importance for human survival. Hemopoietic dysfunction, whether from too much or too little blood cell formation, can cause diseases such as anemia in the case of deficiency or polycythemia in the case of excess. Similarly, AIDS is associated with white blood cell deficiency, while certain types of leukemia, a form of blood cancer, involve the proliferation of abnormal white cells. Much of this information, particularly the process of hematopoiesis, was mysterious until the research of Russian-born hematologist Alexander Maximow clarified its function and the true nature of lymphocytes. **Alexander Maximow** (1874–1928) was born in St. Petersburg and earned his MD in 1896, becoming a professor of histology and embryology. He was awarded a PhD in 1899 for his doctoral dissertation on the pathological regeneration of the testes. He also conducted important experimental work inducing amyloid degeneration of animal liver. In

1903, he became a Russian Army General and in 1919, a professor in the Department of Embryology at St. Petersburg University. In 1922, he fled the Communist Revolution and moved to the US to serve as a professor of anatomy at the University of Chicago, where he taught histology until his death. Maximow died unexpectedly at the peak of his professional career and is buried at Oak Woods Cemetery in Chicago.

For twenty years (1902-1922), Maximow's research focused on the formation of blood and connective tissue. In 1906, he introduced the term "stem cell" for the complete blood-building system, and in 1909, he became internationally renowned for his experimental work that introduced the Unitarian Theory of hematopoiesis, suggesting that all blood cells develop from a common mother stem cell in the bone marrow. He also provided evidence confirming that lymphocytes in blood and lymph nodes are undifferentiated cells. At the same time, he implemented the newly discovered method of tissue culturing, an essential technique for biomedical research in which cells survive and multiply outside the body.

Maximow's two-volume textbook, considered the world's most important reference on histology at the time, was published. His collection of papers at the University of Chicago includes drawings, correspondence, laboratory notes, sketches, and manuscripts of scientific papers and addresses. Maximow is widely regarded as the founder of the hematopoietic stem cell concept, which paved the way for revolutionary treatment strategies such as hematopoietic stem cell transplantation, ushering in a new era in the management of life-threatening blood malignancies.

Demystifying the Genes

The discovery of DNA, the microscopic substance, was made by Swiss physician Friedrich Miescher in 1869 from white blood cells. In 1929, American biochemist Phoebus Levene identified a nucleic acid sugar and proposed that DNA (Deoxy Ribonucleic Acid) consists of a chain of four nucleotide units linked by phosphate groups. In 1933, Belgian biochemist Jean Brachet located DNA within the cell nucleus while studying sea urchin eggs. The landmark Avery-MacLeod-McCarty experiment was conducted in 1944 by three physicians at the Rockefeller Institute in New York City. It identified DNA as the substance responsible for bacterial transformation, overturning the belief that proteins carried genetic information. The experiment marked the beginning of molecular genetics, as later confirmed by scientists. The study was carried out by two Canadian-Americans, **Oswald Avery Jr** (1877-1955) and **Colin MacLeod** (1909-1972), along with their American colleague Maclyn McCarty.

Avery's family emigrated from England to New York City when he was ten years old. He obtained a medical degree in 1904 and spent most of his career at the Rockefeller University Hospital in New York City, becoming one of the first molecular biologists and a pioneer in immunochemistry. The Avery-MacLeod-McCarty experiment was the first in a series of works conducted by Avery and served as a platform for James Watson and Francis Crick to discover the helical structure of DNA, leading to the birth of modern genetics and molecular biology. Despite being nominated for the Nobel Prize multiple times throughout the 1930s, 1940s, and 1950s, Avery and his colleagues did not receive the award, but Avery was honored with a lunar crater named after him.

MacLeod earned his medical degree from McGill University in Montreal in 1932. After moving to New York City in 1934, he joined the Rockefeller Institute and worked closely with Avery on DNA, first as an assistant and later as an associate. Along with Maclyn McCarty, the three demonstrated that DNA is the transforming factor and basis of genes. Later, MacLeod shifted his focus to microbial diseases such as typhus fever, malaria, and cholera. He went on to accept a position as a professor and department chair at New York University before eventually working at the University of Pennsylvania School of Medicine. MacLeod was appointed as a consultant to the US Secretary of War and later became the deputy director of the White House Office of Science and Technology under President John Kennedy in 1963. After Kennedy's assassination, he continued serving as the lead adviser to the White House on policy for the biomedical community under President Johnson. MacLeod was also a member of the first NIH study section on antibiotics and served as an informal advisor to several National Institute of Health Directors, earning membership in the National Academy of Sciences. In 1970, he moved to Oklahoma City to become the president of the Oklahoma Medical Research Foundation, a position he held until his unexpected death while traveling on a layover in London.

Lifesaving Tests

Diphtheria is a severe bacterial infection that affects children, caused by Corynebacterium diphtheriae, which produces a toxin that can lead to enlarged lymph nodes in the neck and swelling in the throat, a condition commonly referred to as "bull neck" that can cause breathing difficulties. In severe cases, a tracheotomy may be necessary to open the airway and allow breathing, and heart failure, paralysis, and even death may occur. In 1904, Ruth Cleveland, the eldest daughter of President Grover Cleveland, died of diphtheria at the age of 12 in Princeton, New Jersey.

In 1927, diphtheria affected 100,000 Americans, resulting in about 10,000 deaths. Although the disease was treatable, it was challenging to determine which patients were predisposed to the disease and required treatment. However, a Hungarian-American pediatrician named **Béla Schick** (1877–1967) developed a susceptibility test that could determine who had been exposed to the disease. The test eventually helped eradicate diphtheria from the US and many parts of the world. Schick was born in Balatonboglár, Hungary, and raised in Graz, Austria. He persuaded his father to allow him to pursue a medical education in pediatrics, rather than joining the family grain merchant business. After completing medical school education in Vienna, he worked at the Children's Clinic in Vienna and became an associate professor of pediatrics at the Medicine Faculty of the University of Vienna in 1902, where he remained until 1923. During his tenure, Schick studied problems of immunity, and with Clemens Pirquet, an Austrian pediatrician, he first coined the term "allergy" as a clinical entity. In 1905, adequate doses of antitoxin for diphtheria became available for disease prevention, and in 1906, Pirquet and Schick described serum sickness in children receiving large quantities of horse-derived antitoxin. A diphtheria vaccine is given to those who have not had prior exposure, but the problem remained of determining who did not have the antibodies and should be given the vaccine.

In 1913, Schick developed the test that was named after him and made him, at the time, a household name in the medical community worldwide. The Schick test involves injecting a small amount (0.1 ml) of diluted diphtheria toxin in the skin of one arm of the person and another heat-inactivated toxin in the other arm as a control. If the patient does not have enough antibodies to fight off the disease, the skin around the injection will become red and swollen for a few days as compared to the control injection, indicating a positive test. If the person has immunity from prior infection, then no swelling or redness will occur, indicating a negative result. The test was created at a time when immunizing agents or vaccines were scarce or not safe. However, as safer toxoids or inactivated toxins became available, susceptibility tests were no longer required.

In 1923, Schick emigrated to the US where he lived the remaining half of his life and directed the Pediatric Department of Mount Sinai Hospital, in New York City. In 1936, he became clinical professor at Columbia University and in 1950 he headed the Pediatric Department of Beth-El Hospital, Brooklyn. While in America helping eradicate diphtheria, Schick made another important advancement in the care of scarlet fever, tuberculosis, and the nutrition for newborns, and children's feeding problems.

A massive campaign was organized by Schick for five years. This campaign included the distribution of 85 million pieces of literature by the Metropolitan Life Insurance Company urging parents to "Save your child from diphtheria." Later, a vaccine was developed to prevent the disease, and as a result, deaths began declining substantially in 1924. Only those who had not been exposed to diphtheria were vaccinated.

Although an effective diphtheria vaccine is available today and given along with pertussis and tetanus vaccines (DPT), sporadic cases are still being reported worldwide, and disease outbreaks are encountered in third world countries as well as in sub-Saharan Africa, India, and Indonesia. In 2015, there were 4,500 cases reported with 5-10% fatalities. **Gerta Ries**, the German-American artist, was commissioned to create sculpted medals as a tribute to Dr. Béla Schick for the Jewish-American Hall of Fame.

Uterine cancer usually develops from the inner lining of the uterus (endometrial cancer 90%), but it can also rarely develop from the muscle wall. In 2010, uterine cancer resulted in 58,000 deaths worldwide. In the US, uterine cancer is most frequently diagnosed among women with a median age of 63, and about 773,000 women were diagnosed with the disease in 2016. About 80% of women with uterine cancer survive five years. If the cancer is localized, the survival rate is 95%, but if there is any spread of the cancer, only 17% survive five years after disease onset.

Vaginal bleeding is a symptom of uterine cancer, but it may also be caused by several other conditions. While a pelvic examination can be helpful, it does not necessarily make the diagnosis. Historically, the dilation and curettage procedure has been used, and it is still being used sometimes for making a definitive diagnosis of uterine cancer. However, it is an invasive procedure that requires anesthesia.

In 1713, an Italian physician named Bernardino Ramazzini made the observation that nuns had a lower incidence of cervical cancer than other women, leading him to assume that sexual intercourse was a risk factor for the disease. Cervical cancer is a type of malignancy that develops in the cervix, which is the lower part of the cervical canal connected to the uterus. It is caused by infection with the human papillomavirus (HPV), which targets the epithelial cells lining the cervix and cervical canal. However, most cases of HPV infection do not progress to cancer. Cervical cancer is the fourth most common type of cancer and the fourth most common cause of cancer-related deaths among women worldwide. In 2012, there were approximately 528,000 cases of cervical cancer globally, resulting in 266,000 deaths. In the US, there were 13,170 new cases of cervical cancer and 4,250 related deaths in 2019. The median age of onset for cervical cancer is 50 years, which is younger than the median age for uterine cancer. In the early stages, there are no symptoms, but later stages may involve vaginal bleeding, pelvic pain, or pain during sexual intercourse. Diagnosis of cervical cancer or pre-cancerous states requires a biopsy of the cervix, which is an invasive procedure.

Early detection is critical for improving survival rates after uterine and cervical cancers. Despite the potential for false results, screening is the best strategy for early diagnosis, especially for women with risk factors. In 1928, a noninvasive screening test was introduced by a Greek immigrant physician named **Georgios Papanikolaou**, which allowed for the diagnosis of both uterine and, more importantly, cervical cancer in the early precancerous stages. Due to widespread use of this screening test, cervical cancer deaths in the US have decreased by approximately 74% in the last 50 years. Papanikolaou **(Fig 24)** was born on the Greek island of Euboea and studied literature, philosophy, languages, and music at the University of Athens. He graduated from the University of Munich medical school in 1904 and served as an army surgeon in the Balkan Wars. In 1913, he emigrated to the US with little money and struggled to make a living, selling carpets, and playing violin in restaurants. Eventually, he was recruited to the Department of Pathology at New York Hospital and the Department of Anatomy at Cornell Medical College, where he focused on examining cancer cells.

In 1920, while working with guinea pigs, Papanikolaou observed that cells shed from the uterine cervix were influenced by hormones. He then used his wife as a volunteer to collect daily vaginal smears, which he examined to determine the stage of her menstrual cycle. Later, he collected cell specimens from women with various gynecological conditions and noticed that he could diagnose the presence of cancer cells by examining pathological smears of exfoliating cervical and uterine cells. His work was not appreciated until the 1950s, when he began using the test to detect aberrant cells that were precursors to cancer. This test became known as the Papanikolaou test or Pap smear and is now used worldwide for the detection and prevention of cervical cancer.

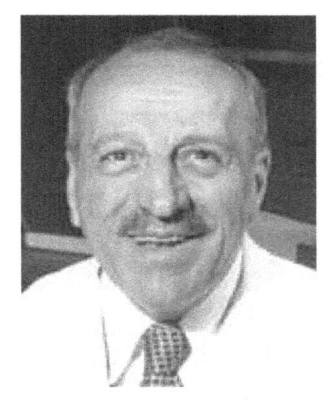

Fig 24. Greek immigrant physician Georgios Papanikolaou the discoverer of the Pap smear. (Samuel Wood Library, Weill Cornell Medicine)

In 1952, the National Cancer Institute launched the largest clinical trial for cancer prevention using the Pap smear. In the United States, screening is recommended as early as age 21, regardless of risk factors, and should be done every three years until the age of 65. Screening may be discontinued after that age if the woman had no abnormal screening results within the previous ten years. Pap test screening every three to five years can reduce cervical cancer incidence by up to 80%.

Papanikolaou was nominated twice for the Nobel Prize but received the Lasker Award in 1950. In 1961, he moved to Miami, Florida, and established a cancer research institute that was named after him. In

1978, Papanikolaou's work was recognized by the US Postal Service with a stamp for early cancer detection.

Men of Hormones Nerves and Syndromes

The endocrine system is made up of various ductless glands scattered throughout the body, which release hormones directly into the bloodstream rather than through ducts. Endocrinology, a branch of medicine, deals with glandular diseases and their respective hormones. One doctor who played a significant role in this field was **Charles Brown-Séquard** (1817–1894), an immigrant physician. He hypothesized that hormones are secreted into the bloodstream to influence distant organs and also described a form of spinal cord injury that was named after him. Born in Mauritius, an African island nation in the Indian Ocean under British rule, Brown-Séquard studied medicine in Paris and eventually moved to the United States, where he taught at the Medical College of Virginia. However, he frequently moved around and worked in various other institutions, such as the National Hospital for the Paralyzed and Epileptic in London and the École de Médecine in Paris.

Brown-Séquard was among the first to examine the physiology of the spinal cord, and his name was immortalized by the description of Brown-Séquard syndrome, a condition he observed after an accidental injury to the spinal cord of sugar cane farmers in Mauritius. This syndrome explains that cutting halfway through the spinal cord results in paralysis and loss of proprioception (the sense of motion) on the same side of the body as the lesion, and loss of pain and temperature sensation on the opposite side of the injury.

Brown-Séquard was an eccentric figure and peripatetic, rarely settling in one place. He returned to Paris and in 1859 went to London to become physician at the National Hospital for the Paralyzed and Epileptic researching and teaching the pathology of the nervous system. In 1864, he returned to the US and was appointed professor of physiology and neuropathology at Harvard medical school. Then he went to France and became a professor at the École de Médecine in Paris, but in 1873 returned to the US and practiced in NY City. Finally, he accepted a position in the Collège de France in Paris where he died.

Brown-Séquard self-experimented at age 72, to rejuvenate sexual competency by subcutaneous injection of extracts of dog and guinea pig testicles. He reported in *The Lancet* that his vigor and feeling of well-being were substantially restored albeit the effects were transient.

Suffering the ridicule of his colleagues, he abandoned the work on the androgens but this experiment at the time was the first attempt to use testosterone to boost men libido but more importantly stimulated subsequent research on the sex hormones. In the 1930s American and European pharmaceutical companies began producing commercially the testosterone hormone to counter the effects of male hypogonadism by improving sexual function and even alleviating symptoms of menopause in women. An estimated 2.3 million American men were receiving androgen hormone therapy in 2013.

Brown-Séquard is considered the father of modern endocrinology, as he was one of the first to postulate the existence of hormones that affect distant organs through the bloodstream. He also discovered the importance of the adrenal gland for life and the connection between its excision and Addison's disease. Despite residing in five countries on three continents and crossing the Atlantic 60 times, Brown-Séquard found time to perform ingenious experiments and write over 500 scientific papers.

The human spinal cord has 31 pairs of nerve roots that become peripheral nerves in the upper or lower limbs. These nerves are either sensory, receiving pain, pressure, touch, and temperature sensations, or motor, sending electrical impulses that cause muscles to contract and move body parts. Nerve compression occurs when nerve roots or peripheral nerves are compressed in a confined anatomical space, causing symptoms that vary in severity and duration. These symptoms may be mild or moderate, causing discomfort, numbness, tingling, clumsiness of movement, and weakness, or severe, causing sensation loss and muscle paralysis. Nerve root compression produces radiculopathy, or pain radiating to the neck or lower back. Examples of nerve compressions in the upper extremity are, carpal tunnel syndrome, cubital tunnel syndrome, and thoracic outlet syndrome. Carpal tunnel syndrome is the most common nerve compression disorder, affecting the median nerve in the hand and causing nocturnal symptoms that disturb sleep and compromise the ability to use the hand in daily activities. Most cases of carpal tunnel syndrome can be treated conservatively, but chronic and severe cases require hand surgery. The radial nerve is responsible for extending the elbow, wrist, fingers, and thumb and terminates in a superficial sensory branch that supplies sensation to the back and side of the wrist and hand. Compression of the radial nerve in the arm may cause paralysis of the muscles responsible for elbow, wrist, and hand movement. Although rare, compression of the sensory component of the radial nerve in the wrist may occur, and known as Wartenberg syndrome, named after the Russian-American neurologist **Robert Wartenberg** (1887-1956), who identified this nerve compression and other nerve disorders.

Wartenberg was born in Grodno, old Lithuania, and studied medicine at the University of Rostock in Germany, graduating in 1919. He became a professor of neurology at the University of Freiburg until 1935 when he escaped the Nazi regime and emigrated to San Francisco to become a professor at the University of California. In 1925, he became a Travelling Fellow of the Rockefeller Foundation, visiting the United Kingdom, France, and US centers, including Boston, where he worked with Harvey Cushing, a neurosurgeon who trained at Johns Hopkins Hospital and wrote a biography of William Osler. Wartenberg wrote over 150 papers in German and English and two important books, translated into many languages, on clinical neurology and nerve reflexes and signs.

He is also known for the Wartenberg sign, which occurs in ulnar nerve compression and paralysis commonly seen among cyclists. This condition causes the small finger to acquire an abnormal abduction posture that compromises hand function. Additionally, he developed the Wartenberg neurological wheel, a device that systematically rotates over the skin to test skin sensitivity. The Wartenberg head-dropping test is encountered among Parkinson's disease patients. Cheiralgia paresthetica, also known as Wartenberg syndrome, can be caused by the application of pressure on the wrist, such as wearing a tight wristwatch or bracelet, causing compression of the sensory part of the radial nerve with hand numbness and pain. It can also be caused by constricting handcuffs, a condition known as handcuff neuropathy, which can be associated with carpal tunnel syndrome.

Wartenberg helped found the American Academy of Neurology in 1948 and continues to be commemorated by this Academy's annual Robert Wartenberg Lecture. He was an honorary member of neurological societies in several countries. Wartenberg adopted a method of diagnosing and treating patients with minimum laboratory tests, avoiding invasive and expensive procedures. This practice is still relevant today in light of the staggering cost of healthcare.

Scrutinizing the Cells

Looking under a microscope in 1839, two Germans a physician Theodor Schwann and botanist Matthias Schleiden found that plants and animals are made of cells, concluding that cells are a common founding entity thus established the cell theory; meaning the cell is the basic structural and functional unit of life forms. Schwann also identified the Schwann cells, a crucial component of peripheral nerves. Although plant and animal cells are visible only under a light microscope, their dimensions are measured in micrometers or microns, which is one thousandth of a millimeter or one millionth of a meter. For instance, a human red blood cell is approximately 5 microns in diameter while a white blood cell measures about 30 microns. The human body contains an estimated 37 trillion cells, each consists of a cell membrane that encloses a nucleus suspended in the cytoplasmic liquid. The cytoplasm also contains mitochondria, vesicles, Golgi apparatus, and the rough endoplasmic reticulum. These cellular constituents are best viewed using an electron microscope. However, the breakthrough method of cell fractionation was necessary to identify them, which allowed the isolation of each cellular component and biochemical analysis while preserving their individual function. The innovator of this method was Belgium-American **Albert Claude** (1899 –1983).

Born in Longlier, Belgium, Claude witnessed his mother's battle with and death from breast cancer and began working as a bellboy at the age of twelve. He later volunteered in the British Intelligence Service during WWI and eventually pursued his interest in cells, particularly cancer research, while studying at the University of Liège in Belgium. In 1929, Claude was granted a fellowship to conduct research in the United States, where he joined the Rockefeller Institute in New York. One year later, he developed the technique of cell fractionation, which revolutionized the field of scientific investigation by allowing the isolation of cellular components and their biochemical analysis while preserving their function. With this method, Claude discovered the agent of the Rous sarcoma and became the first person to use the electron microscope in biology. He later succeeded, with the Canadian-American **Keith Porter** (1912-1997), in obtaining electron micrographs of cultured fibroblasts, showing a lace-like endoplasmic reticulum. Claude became a US citizen in 1941 and a professor at the Rockefeller University as well as the University of Louvain, where he spent the rest of his retirement in Brussels.

For his pioneering work, Claude received many awards including the Louisa Gross Horwitz Prize (1970), together with George Palade and Keith Porter; the Paul Ehrlich and Ludwig Darmstaedter Prize

(1971); and the 1974 Nobel Prize in Physiology or Medicine with his student the Romanian-American cell biologist **George Palade** (1912-2008) and Christian de Duve. Like Claude Palade was a physician and cell biologist. He was Romanian-born and emigrated to the US in 1946, where he joined Claude at the Rockefeller Institute. In addition to the Nobel Prize Palade won many awards and was described as "the most influential cell biologist ever."

Machines that Save Lives

The kidney is an essential organ that plays a critical role in maintaining overall health. Chronic kidney disease, which causes loss of kidney function or renal failure, can present with symptoms such as leg swelling, fatigue, vomiting, loss of appetite, and confusion. If left untreated, kidney malfunction can increase the risk of heart complications, cause uremia, and ultimately lead to seizures, coma, and death. Triggers of this condition include diabetes, high blood pressure, nephritis (chronic kidney inflammation), and congenital polycystic kidney disease. In the US, renal failure affects almost 750,000 people every year.

For severe kidney disease, a kidney transplant is a viable treatment option. This procedure involves replacing the affected kidney with another one from a compatible donor, either a live volunteer or a recently deceased person. In 1933, Ukrainian surgeon Yuriy Vorony attempted the first human kidney transplant by placing a kidney from a dead donor into the patient's thigh. Unfortunately, the organ was rejected due to incompatibility, and the patient died two days later. In 1950, Richard Lawler successfully performed the first kidney transplant on a woman with polycystic kidney disease in Evergreen Park, Illinois. However, the donated kidney was rejected ten months later because immunosuppressive therapy was unavailable at that time.

In 2018, over 100,000 patients in the US were on a waiting list for a kidney transplant, but only around 21,000 donor organs were available for transplantation. Not every patient with renal failure is eligible for a kidney transplant. For those who are not, kidney dialysis is the only other widely available treatment option. Dialysis involves using an external filtration machine to remove excess water and toxins from the blood or abdomen. It can be a temporary treatment for patients awaiting a donor kidney transplant or a permanent measure for those whom a transplant is not possible. Before 1913, kidney dialysis did not exist. It was not until two physicians, Canadian-born Rowntree, and Dutch-born Kolff, worked together to invent the first prototypical artificial kidney machine in the US. This was followed by the development of the first practical lifesaving kidney dialysis machine.

Leonard Rowntree (1883–1959) was born in London, Ontario, and graduated from the University of Western Ontario medical school in 1905. After moving to Camden, New Jersey, at the suggestion of his physician uncle, he attended a lecture by William Osler, who recommended him to work with pharmacologist John Abel at Johns Hopkins Hospital in 1907. Rowntree began working with Abel in 1909 and learned from him about phenol, a red dye used to develop the Rowntree-Geraghty test, which was the first kidney function analysis to estimate overall blood flow through the kidney. This test was used for almost a century before it was replaced by more contemporary methods.

With Abel's help, Rowntree **(Fig 25)** developed the first artificial kidney machine in 1913 and successfully tested it on animals. Later, Rowntree was able to centrifuge blood by separating plasma from blood cells, a procedure that Abel later called "plasmapheresis". The concept of the artificial kidney was later adopted by the immigrant American Kolff, who in 1943 developed the first workable dialysis machine worldwide.

In 1915, Rowntree became the head of medicine at the University of Minnesota in Rochester. After suffering from a life-threatening

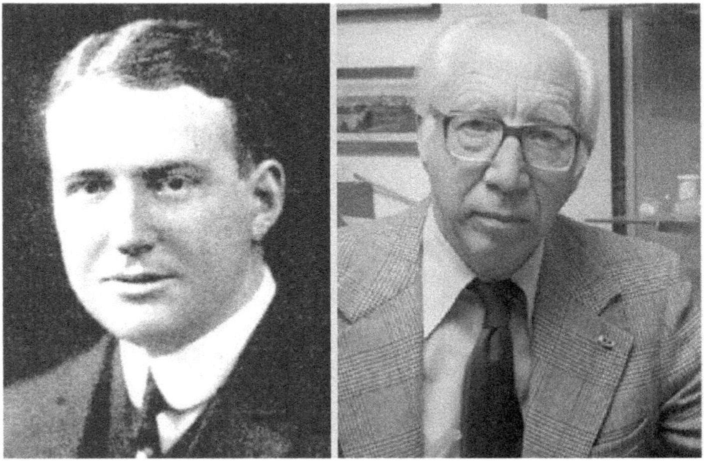

Fig 25. Immigrant physicians Leonard Rowntree (left) and Willem Kolff (right), inventors of kidney dialysis system. Kolff is also considered the Father of Artificial Organs. (Medical Society and U J Willard Marriott Library Utah University)

perforated gastric ulcer in 1918, he had surgery by William Mayo, who saved his life. In 1920, Rowntree was appointed Professor and Head of Medicine of the Mayo Foundation in Minnesota, where he recruited more than a dozen researchers who became known as the "Rowntree Group" to conduct clinical investigations while he worked on endocrine and kidney disease and blood research. In 1923, he collaborated with Osborne to use iodide as a tool for imaging the anatomy of the kidney and urinary tract, known as intravenous pyelogram, which is still being used today.

In 1932, after thirteen years, Rowntree left Mayo Clinic for a less demanding role in his adopted hometown of Philadelphia, becoming Director of the Philadelphia Institute for Medical Research. During World War II, he volunteered and was appointed head of the Medical Service of the Selective Service System. After the war, he retired with his wife to Florida and helped set up the University of Miami School of Medicine in 1952 but continued to be active until his passing.

For his service in the armed forces, Rowntree was awarded a Presidential Citation in 1946 by President Harry Truman. He was elected an honorary member of the Harvey Club of London, awarded an honorary Doctor of Science degree from the University of Western Ontario, and won the Banting Medal of the American Diabetes Association. No record could be found of Rowntree becoming an American citizen. Whether he applied for citizenship is unclear, but what was clear is that he adopted the US as his country and spent the last fifty-three years of his life innovating and serving his country.

Willem Kolff (1911–2009) was a Dutch physician who completed his medical education and internal medicine training at Leiden University in 1938. After watching a young patient slowly dying of chronic kidney failure, he was motivated to conduct research to find a treatment for renal failure.

In 1943, Kolff created the first prototype dialyzer based on Rowntree's artificial kidney, which was intended to remove waste products and excess fluid from the blood of patients with kidney failure. After two years of failed attempts and refinements, he finally succeeded in treating his first patient with kidney failure using his hemodialysis machine. This patient was a 67-year-old woman, whose life was saved, making it the first functioning artificial kidney.

Kolff **(Fig 25)** donated his artificial kidney machines to hospitals in Europe and one to Dutch-American physician **Isidore Snapper** at Mount Sinai Hospital in New York City. This machine was used to perform the first human dialysis in the US in 1948, under the supervision of Drs. Alfred Fishman and Irving Kroop.

In 1950, Kolff emigrated to the US, where he worked at the Cleveland Clinic, Ohio, and was involved in the development of the heart-lung machine, which maintains cardiac and pulmonary functions during heart surgery. This pump-oxygenator machine was useful and helped make open-heart surgery a feasible technique. Kolff then practiced at Brigham and Women's Hospital in Boston, where he improved his dialysis machine and developed the first production machine, the Kolff-Brigham Artificial Kidney. Lastly, he settled in Salt Lake City in 1967, where he became head of the Division of Artificial Organs and the Institute for Biomedical Engineering at the University of Utah. There he shifted his focus to the development of an implantable artificial heart. After a series of attempts and working with a team of researchers and physicians, the final model was first implanted in 1982 in Barney Clark, who survived for four months.

Kolff is considered the Father of Artificial Organs and one of the most important physicians of the 20th century. He was a pioneer of hemodialysis and the developer of the kidney machine in 1943 and 1945. The machine, which has carried his name since its invention, has saved the lives of millions of patients with acute or chronic kidney failure. His work on the artificial heart inspired others to refine the invention and ushered in an age of organ transplantation.

Kolff received more than 12 honorary doctorates from universities around the world and more than 120 international awards, including the Cameron Prize for Therapeutics from the University of Edinburgh, the Golden Plate Award of the American Academy of Achievement, the Harvey Prize, AMA Scientific Achievement Award, the Japan Prize, Albert Lasker Award, and the Russ Prize. In 1990, Life Magazine included him in a list of the 100 Most Important Persons of the 20th Century. Robert Jarvik, who worked in Kolff's laboratory at the University of Utah, credited Kolff with inspiring him to develop the first permanent artificial heart.

Vaccine and Nicotine

In the early 1950s, polio viral infection outbreaks were a major concern worldwide, and in the US, the disease caused over 15,000 cases of childhood limb paralysis. However, polio vaccine, which prevents poliomyelitis and provides permanent immunity, has been successful in eliminating the disease from most of the world, with the exception of recent cases among unvaccinated people. Two physicians, Jonas Salk and **Albert Sabin**, are credited with developing two different polio vaccines, one inactivated and the other weakened. Salk's inactivated vaccine, which is given by injection, was the first successful vaccine released in 1955, but it did not prevent the initial intestinal infection, and administering it by injection is challenging for children.

Sabin, who was born in Białystok, Russian Empire (Poland) to Jewish parents, became a naturalized US citizen in 1930 after graduating from high school in Paterson, New Jersey. He studied virology and received a medical degree from New York University Medical School, then trained in internal medicine, pathology, and surgery at Bellevue Hospital in New York City. Sabin's interest in infectious diseases led him to join the Rockefeller Institute, and in 1939 he moved to Cincinnati Children's Hospital in Ohio. During World War II, he helped develop a vaccine against Japanese encephalitis while serving in the US Army Medical Corps, and he worked at several medical facilities in South Carolina, Washington DC, and Cincinnati.

With the increasing threat of polio, researchers like Salk and Sabin sought to find a vaccine to combat the disease. Sabin, while working in Ohio, demonstrated that the poliovirus attacked the intestines before spreading to the central nervous system, and he developed his attenuated oral vaccine in 1954, which blocked the virus from being absorbed into the bloodstream through the intestine. The earliest recipients of this vaccine were Sabin himself, his family, and colleagues. Between 1956 and 1960, he collaborated with Russian scientists to perfect the oral vaccine, which was used internationally among 100 million people before it was approved in the US in 1960, when mass immunizations of school children began. The Sabin oral vaccine, which was easier to administer to children with sugar cubes, became more popular than the Salk injection route, and the effects of the oral vaccine lasted longer, becoming the predominant method of vaccination.

As a result of the success of the vaccines, the number of polio cases in the US fell rapidly to a handful in the 1970s. In 1988, the "Global Polio Eradication Initiative" was launched, which nearly eradicated the disease in 2016 when the number of cases worldwide was reduced by 99.99%. Sabin became a philanthropist and was honored with numerous awards, including having a hospital, a street, and a convention center named after him in Cincinnati.

Ernst Wynder (1922-1999) was born to Jewish parents in Prussia, and his family escaped Nazi rule to the United States in 1938. Wynder attended New York University and later joined the army during World War II, where he was assigned to a psychological warfare unit monitoring German newscasts due to his German-speaking skills. After the war, he received his medical degree from Washington University in St. Louis in 1950 and began working at the Sloan-Kettering Institute for Cancer Research. Wynder dedicated his career to cancer and chronic disease prevention as a researcher, educator, and activist.

Wynder's early work with research collaborator Evarts Graham on smoking's role in causing lung cancer was groundbreaking. Their epidemiologic study was published in the Journal of the American Medical Association, providing significant scientific evidence that smoking was a contributory cause of lung cancer. Wynder and Graham also conducted a study on the impact of cigarette tar from tobacco smoke on the skin of mice, which caused malignant tumors. Throughout his career, Wynder published nearly 800 papers primarily on the epidemiology of various cancers including those affecting the breast, bladder, larynx, colon, stomach, ovary, prostate, and kidney.

Despite years of criticism from the tobacco industry, Wynder remained steadfast in his efforts. He left Sloan-Kettering and founded the American Health Foundation in 1969, where he served as medical director and launched the Preventive Medicine Journal with himself as editor. At the time of his death, the foundation employed about 200 researchers from various fields such as medicine, public health, biology, chemistry, nutrition, and behavioral science. In recognition of his achievements, he was awarded the Robert Koch Prize.

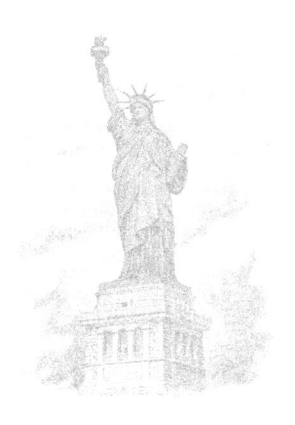

CHAPTER 8

Physicians in Specialized Fields

Since Galen's time, Roman doctors have chosen to specialize, becoming either clinicians or surgeons. During the 19th century, informal specializations began to evolve. Medical specialty is now a practice that focuses on a defined group of patients or diseases, where after completing medical school, physicians engage in further medical education emphasizing a specific branch by completing a multiple-year residency. After residency, some choose to *subspecialize* by undertaking a fellowship. Specialties may be organ-based, such as ophthalmology or urology; others are age-based, such as pediatrics or geriatrics; and some are technology-centered, like radiology or endoscopy. Then, there are some specialties which stand apart from any given categories, like forensic medicine or rehabilitation. The Accreditation Council for Graduate Medical Education (ACGME) is a private not-for-profit organization that sets the standards for all US graduate medical education. In the academic year 2021–22, there were approximately 871 ACGME-accredited institutions sponsoring approximately 12,740 residency and fellowship programs in 182 specialties and subspecialties.

Of all those many specialties, four are discussed here along with the impact that immigrants have had on them. Two are organ-based, orthopedic surgery and cardiology; one is technology-based, ultrasound; and the last is psychiatry, which is an abstract field that treats mental and behavioral disorders.

Orthopedic Surgery and Immigrant Orthopedic Surgeons

The ancient history of orthopedic surgery can be traced back to the Stone Age, when crude amputations were performed. Ancient Egyptians used splints, which were discovered in mummies for treating fractures of thigh and forearm bones and are dated back to about 3000 BCE. Some splints were made of bamboo and reed, padded with linen. Crutches were also used by ancient Egyptians, as depicted in a carving on one Egyptian tomb in 2830 BCE. The Shoshone Indians, who existed around 700-2000 BCE, made splints for injured limbs out of rawhide. The Greeks, and later Arabs, had a great deal of orthopedic knowledge of fractures and dislocations. The French Ambroise Paré lived in a time when physicians considered surgery beneath their dignity and left it to the less respected barber-surgeons. His avant-garde treatments mentioned earlier in this book raised the status of surgeons. Paré used prostheses for amputated limbs, including a prosthetic hand. In the 19th and 20th centuries, rapid developments in treating orthopedic infections ensued.

The introduction of novel technology, particularly the discovery of X-ray by German Wilhelm Rontgen was crucial for diagnosing and treating orthopedic conditions. In October 1895, Rontgen placed his wife Anna's hand between a tube that emitted invisible rays and a photographic plate. The skeletal anatomy of her hand and her wedding ring were visible on the plate, which Rontgen called X-ray. When Rontgen's wife saw her hand X-ray, she shook in horror, thinking that X-ray was a harbinger of death. In 1914, X-rays were used on the battlefields of WWI. In 1926, American geneticist Nobel laureate Herman Muller demonstrated that X-rays could cause cell mutation, with the potential danger of overexposure to radiation. In 1946, Muller was awarded the Nobel Prize in Physiology or Medicine for "the discovery that mutations can be induced by X-rays." In 1902, a French couple, Pierre and Marie Curie, were able to harness more powerful X-ray energy from the new element that Marie called radium, which later became the basis for radiation therapy used for cancer treatment. Today's advanced imaging includes CT (computerized tomography) scans, MRI (magnetic resonance imaging), and PET (Positron Emission Tomography) scans.

The human musculoskeletal system is made up of muscles and their tendons, bones and their cartilage, and joints with their ligaments, all of which provide the body with form, support, stability, and movement. The orthopedic surgery specialty manages a wide range of diseases and injuries of the musculoskeletal system. The term "orthopedics" originates from two words: "orthos," meaning "straight," and "paidios," meaning "child," which was coined by the French physician Nicolas Andry in his book titled Orthopédie (1741) and meant the correction of musculoskeletal deformities in children. Thus, some consider Andry as the founder of the orthopedic surgery specialty. Others believe the true father of orthopedics is Swiss surgeon Jean Andre Vedal (1740-1791) because he established the first orthopedic institute in Orbe, Switzerland, in 1780, which was a hospital dedicated to the treatment of children's skeletal deformities; the building now serves as a museum. The earliest gets the credit.

The British physician Percival Pott published *Some Few Remarks upon Fractures and Dislocations* in 1769, describing deformities resulting from tuberculosis of the spine, a disease that now bears his name. Pott was the first to establish in 1775 the association between cancer and environmental factors when he described a chimneysweeper with cancer of the scrotum from soot as a carcinogen.

The French surgeon Guillaume Dupuytren published a book titled *On the Injuries and Disease of the Bone* in 1847. The Welsh physician Hugh Owen Thomas (1834-1891) and his nephew Robert Jones have been called in modern times "the Fathers of Orthopedic Surgery" for setting and splinting fractures. The German surgeon Gerhard Küntscher (1900-1972) launched the use of metallic nails, K-wires, for treating long bone fractures at a time when patients were treated with traction and lengthy hospital stays. In 1962, English surgeon John Charnley performed the first hip replacement surgery.

In the US, orthopedic surgery has benefited greatly from wartime experiences, leading to increased proficiency in treating open wounds and limb amputations. Early American pioneer orthopedic surgeons introduced innovative treatment techniques that are still in use today. For example, Russell Hibbs (1869-1932) treated joint deformities in adults and children in New York by fusing or mending joints, including spine deformities; a society was formed in 1947 in his name. In 1940, Austin Moore (1899-1963) performed a hip replacement using a cobalt-chrome alloy Vitallium prosthesis that was named after him for the treatment of hip fractures. In 1946, Sterling Bunnell established the American Society for Surgery of the Hand, the oldest and largest hand surgery organization. Don O'Donoghue, a native of Oklahoma, was instrumental in founding the American Orthopedic Society for Sports Medicine in 1972, and the specialty concerned with treating athletic injuries.

The American Academy of Orthopedic Surgeons was established in 1933 by a group of founders, with Edwin Ryerson serving as its first president in 1932. Under the Academy's umbrella today, there are 23 Orthopedic Musculoskeletal Specialty Societies concerned with different areas, including hand, elbow and shoulder, foot and ankle, hip and knee, spine, trauma, tumor, sports, research, and rehabilitation. With over 39,000 members, the AAOS is the world's largest medical organization of musculoskeletal specialists. Orthopedic surgery is one of the most sought-after surgical specialties in the US, with medical school graduates training for five years to become orthopedic surgeons.

Countless immigrant surgeons have had a remarkable influence on the orthopedic surgery specialty in the US. Since the early 18th century, they have brought knowledge from abroad and developed it in their new country, passing it on to modern medical communities and favorably impacting patient care and the professional careers of today's orthopedic surgeons globally. Some were instrumental in medical education or establishing new surgical disciplines and specialty societies. Here, we will only acknowledge those who made paramount contributions. One of those was the German-born surgeon **William Detmold**, whose story was told earlier, and who served in the Civil War, introducing orthopedic surgery as a specialty to the US.

Before the turn of the 20th century, children suffering from flaccid paralysis of poliomyelitis, spastic paralysis of cerebral palsy, and congenital spine deformity of scoliosis had limited treatment options. However, in the early 1900s, surgery began to play a crucial role in alleviating their suffering and improving their quality of life. Orthopedic surgeon **Arthur Steindler** (1878–1959), who was a leading authority in the field, offered special care for these children using novel techniques that surgeons have continued to use for the last 75 years. Steindler was born in a small town in the Austria-Hungarian Empire (Czech Republic) in 1878 and studied in Prague. He graduated from the University of Vienna Medical School in 1902 and emigrated to the US in 1907, where he worked at St Luke's Hospital, Chicago (1907-10) before moving to Iowa, where he settled permanently. He was first appointed as a Professor of Orthopedic Surgery at Drake University, Des Moines in 1915 and then became a Professor of Orthopedic Surgery in Iowa City at the State University College of Medicine. He retired in 1949 but continued working at the Mercy Hospital for several years. Steindler became an American citizen in 1914.

During his professional career, Steindler (**Fig 26**) founded the clinical and academic Orthopedic Surgery programs at the University of Iowa. He also established a statewide program to provide medical care for indigent patients, many of whom were children crippled by polio, tuberculosis, cerebral palsy, scoliosis, and congenital deformities. Steindler acquired an encyclopedic knowledge of orthopedic surgery, which he shared with residents and colleagues. He made major contributions and advancements in the entire range of musculoskeletal disorders. He introduced procedures for the treatment of scoliosis and devised several innovative techniques to restore movements of paralyzed muscles in the upper and lower extremities, some of which are still being used today. Steindler published extensively and wrote several books, including *Reconstructive Surgery of the Upper Extremity* (1923), *Diseases and Deformities of the Spine and Thorax* (1929), *Orthopedic Operations* (1940), *Kinesiology of the Human Body* (1955), and *Lectures on the Interpretation of Pain in Orthopedic Practice* (1959). He served as President of the American Orthopedic Association, an antecedent to the American Academy of Orthopedic Surgeons. Steindler was a friend of Don O'Donoghue, who was on the faculty of the orthopedic surgery department of Oklahoma University, and he told stories about how respected and revered Steindler was in the US and internationally. The "Steindler flexroplasty," an effective technique for restoring motion and function of the paralyzed elbow and upper extremity, was used throughout the writer's entire professional career.

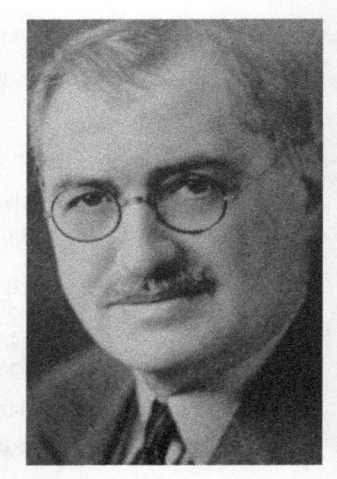

Fig 26. Austrian-American orthopedic surgeon Arthur Steindler, pioneered surgery for children with paralysis, poliomyelitis, cerebral palsy, and congenital limb deformities including scoliosis of the spine. (Who's who in orthopedics)

Osteoporosis is a widespread health issue that affects the elderly, causing fragility fractures of the spine, hip, and wrist, leading to increased morbidity and mortality in the population. While the incidence of hip fractures has decreased over the past 40 years due to better lifestyle choices, studies from the early 2000s revealed that about 30% of older individuals with hip fractures will die within a year, not to mention the severe consequences for those who survive and the financial burden on communities for care. A century ago, the negative impact of these fractures was even greater due to the lack of appropriate treatment, resulting in bed confinement until the fracture healed or the patient passed away. However, an immigrant orthopedic surgeon, **Marius Smith-Petersen** (1886-1953), invented a device to fix hip fractures, allowing the patient to ambulate without confinement, considerably improving their chances of survival and reducing suffering.

Smith-Petersen was born in Grimstad, Norway, to a wealthy and prominent Norwegian family as the youngest of four sons. At the age of sixteen, he and his mother emigrated to the US and settled in Milwaukee, Wisconsin, where he attended high school, college, and medical school. Smith-Petersen transferred from the University of Wisconsin to Harvard Medical School in Cambridge, Massachusetts, where he earned his degree in 1914. He remained in the Boston area for the rest of his life, completing his orthopedic surgery training at Massachusetts General Hospital and ascending the ranks from instructor to clinical professor and Chief of Orthopedic Service (1929-46).

In 1925, Smith-Petersen introduced the three-flanged steel nail that stabilized hip fractures at the neck of the femur, hastening recovery and decreasing mortality rates. His innovation gained him an international reputation for his hip fracture nailing technique. Smith-Petersen also developed other groundbreaking surgical methods, including hip-mold arthroplasty in 1923, which used an implant to treat hip joint arthritis, originally made of glass but later replaced with a bell-shaped

Vitallium cup, which became the precursor to today's hip joint replacement. Additionally, he used osteotomy to correct spinal deformities and continuous irrigation to treat bone infections.

Smith-Petersen died of a heart attack shortly after performing a successful hip replacement operation on Arthur Godfrey, a famous television talk-show host at the time. He was a consultant to the Surgeon General (1942-45) and was awarded the Grand Cross of the Order of St. Olav by the King of Norway. As an orthopedic resident in Baltimore, I was trained using the original Smith-Petersen device for treating adult hip fractures and a modified Smith-Petersen hip nail technique for treating slipped femoral epiphysis in children. Today, screws are used to fix hip fractures, designed as a modification of the Smith-Petersen device. Moreover, throughout my professional career, I have occasionally used his continuous irrigation method for treating bone infections.

Dwarfism, also known as short stature, is a congenital disorder characterized by upper and lower limb deformities. This condition has affected humanity for millennia and was even reported among ancient Egyptians. Musculoskeletal anomalies, such as knee deformities likely caused by polio and humpbacks possibly caused by tuberculosis of the spine, have been documented in mummies and depicted in drawings on Pharaohs' tombs. In fact, a recent X-ray of an Egyptian mummy revealed a primitive prosthesis placed on a congenital amputation of the forearm. Interestingly, congenital deformities associated with dwarfism were once considered divine attributes granted to humans by the gods, and dwarfs even attained high ranks in Pharaohs' courts.

Today, children from all walks of life, regardless of socioeconomic status, may experience congenital musculoskeletal differences of the hand and upper extremities. Fortunately, orthopedic and hand surgeons have made significant progress in correcting these deformities, thanks in part to knowledge inherited from pioneer surgeons in the early 19th and 20th centuries. One such surgeon was **Hamper**

Kelikian (1899-1983), an immigrant from the Ottoman Empire who settled in Chicago in 1920 to escape the Armenian Genocide. After studying at Rush Medical College, Kelikian became an orthopedic surgeon and served as chief orthopedic surgeon and lieutenant colonel at the 297th General Hospital. He specialized in pediatric orthopedic surgery with an emphasis on congenital deformities and even treated children who developed congenital upper extremity phocomelia during the thalidomide tragedy. His book, "Congenital Deformities of the Hand and Forearm" (1974), was one of the earliest textbooks written in English on the subject of hand deformities and their surgical treatments, and it became an important reference for many surgeons for generations. Kelikian also performed several surgical procedures on veteran Bob Dole between 1947 and 1953 to save and restore his arm function. Interestingly, Kelikian never charged Armenians for his treatments.

Kelikian's contributions to the field of orthopedic surgery were widely recognized, and he received many accolades throughout his career. For instance, while serving in the US Army, Kelikian received a citation and a medal from President Harry Truman. He was also invited to visit Lebanon in 1966, where he was awarded the Order of the National Cedars of Lebanon by Lebanese President Charles Helou. In 1969, Kelikian was appointed to President Nixon's Task Force for the Disabled.

Adrian Flatt (1921-2017) was another immigrant orthopedic surgeon who dedicated his career to teaching residents and fellows and treating children with congenital upper extremity and hand differences in the US. He served as president of the American Society for Surgery of the Hand. Besides his immense contributions to the field of orthopedic surgery, Flatt is also known for his epic casting and bronze coating of the hands of famous individuals and for establishing a hand exhibit in Dallas at Baylor Hospital featuring a collection of more than 120 hands, including those of US presidents **(Fig 27)**. Besides Flatt,

Graham Lister was a Scottish immigrant plastic surgeon that also became president of the same hand society.

Throughout history, leprosy has been viewed as a highly infectious, dreadful, and disfiguring disease. Some even believed it to be a curse

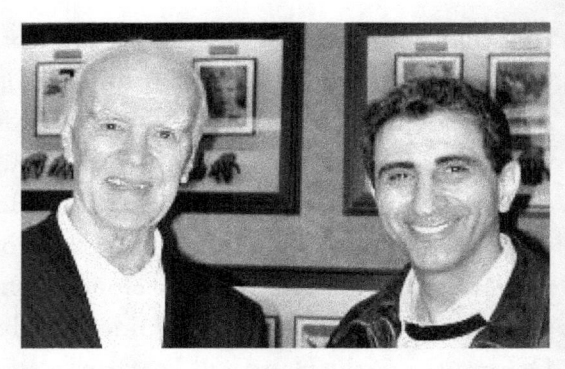

Fig 27. Immigrant pioneer orthopedic surgeon Adrian Flatt (left) with this author at Baylor Hospital Museum in Dallas, where Flatt's collection of hand molds are hosted, 2001.

from God for sinners, and lepers were often ostracized by society and placed in leper colonies. Leprosy is caused by a slow-growing bacterium (Mycobacterium leprae) from the tuberculosis family, which was identified by the Norwegian physician Gerhard Hansen in 1873. In his efforts to further understand the disease, Hansen even inoculated a woman's eye with the bacteria without her permission in 1880, causing her to develop an eye infection.

Hansen's disease, also known as leprosy, is communicable through the lining of the mouth and nose and can affect the nerves, skin, and eyes. If left untreated, the disease can cause nerve damage, resulting in paralysis of the hands and feet, as well as loss of pain and touch sensations. Patients may experience spontaneous amputation of their toes and fingers due to repeated injuries that are not felt as painful. The disease can also cause skin rash, ulceration, infection, and blindness.

Although the geographic origin of the disease is unclear, the oldest documented evidence of leprosy comes from skeletal remains dating back to 2500-2000 BCE in India. Although leprosy existed in Europe as early as 400 BCE, it became widespread in that continent during the medieval period, with 19,000 leprosy hospitals established by 1200. While the prevalence of leprosy globally has declined over the past four decades due to the introduction of anti-tuberculous drug therapy, it remains endemic in several states of India and continues to be a public health challenge in developing countries.

Leprosy was once feared as a highly contagious and destructive disease that could be transmitted by mere touch. However, today we understand that it is less transmissible and severe cases can be treated with surgery. This knowledge is largely gifted by one person; thanks to orthopedic hand surgeon, **Paul Brand** (1914-2003), who dedicated his entire professional career to studying the disease and treating the limbs of leprosy patients in India. Born to missionary parents in India, Brand completed his medical studies at University College Hospital in London during WWII and earned his surgical qualifications while working as a casualty surgeon during the London Blitz. In 1946, he joined the staff of the Christian Medical College and Hospital in Vellore, India.

Brand's research into the reasons behind the deformities developing among patients with Hansen's disease, which was prevalent in India, concluded that the deformities result from a lack of pain and are not directly caused by the bacteria. This dispelled the stigma associated with the disease within the medical community and among the public. Brand established a center in Vellore where he examined and surgically treated many leprosy patients. In 1966, he moved to the United States and took up the position of Chief of the Rehabilitation Branch at the National Hansen's Disease Center in Carville, Louisiana, where he worked for 20 years. Brand pioneered tendon transfer surgery to restore the function of paralytic hands and upper limbs, as well as serial casting as a rehabilitation technique for improving hand deformities. He also conceived the idea of designing a special shoe to help leprosy patients with foot deformities to walk more easily. After retiring, Brand moved to Seattle, Washington, where he passed away. Brand received many awards and served as the President of the Leprosy Mission International. In addition to his many scientific publications, he wrote two books for the general public with Philip Yancey: *In His Image* (1987) and *The Gift of Pain* (1997). A biography of Brand, *Ten Fingers for God*

(1996), was written by Dorothy Clarke Wilson and Philip Yancey.

Brand's extensive knowledge of musculoskeletal mechanics, surgical treatments of the upper extremities, and rehabilitation techniques had an immeasurable influence on the careers of numerous surgeons worldwide, including myself. I was fortunate enough to have met and learned from Doctor Brand, who was my guest lecturer in 1995 at the annual meeting of the American Society for Surgery of the Hand (**Fig 28**). During his lecture, he spoke about his volunteer work in India and how he innovated by making splints out of aluminum from a crashed airplane's fuselage, which allowed crippled children with paralytic legs to walk with the aid of these splints. He also asked his assistant to design rocker-bottom shoes that helped leprosy patients walk comfortably without putting pressure on their foot ulcers. Lucille Travis wrote a book, *Paul Brand: The Shoe that Love Made* (2014), which tells the story of that shoe. Paul Brand was a compassionate, philanthropic, and skilled surgeon whose legacy will undoubtedly last.

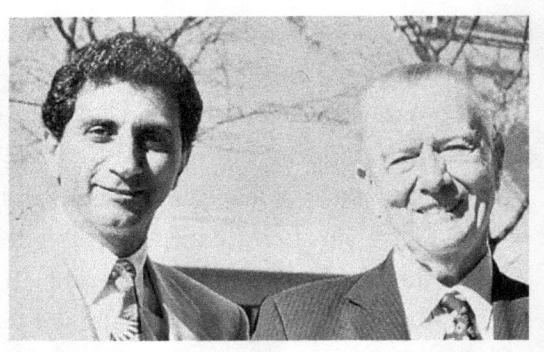

Fig 28. India-born iconic surgeon and humanitarian Paul Brand (right) while hosted by this author (left) during ASSH meeting. Brand dispelled the dogma that leprosy is highly contagious and was the first to operate on its patients, 1994.

Father Damien, a Roman Catholic priest from Belgium, led a ministry from 1873 until his death in 1889 in the Kingdom of Hawai'i, where he cared for people with leprosy living in government-mandated medical quarantine in a settlement on Moloka'i. Despite contracting leprosy from his patients, Father Damien continued to serve the colony until he succumbed to the disease.

Clubfoot is a congenital birth defect where both feet are rotated inward and downward—it is an ancient condition that has been documented throughout history. Without treatment, the foot remains permanently twisted, and the patient walks on ankles and sides of the feet with a severely disabling abnormal gait. According to the World Health Organization, around 100,000 babies worldwide are born annually with clubfoot. However, treatment of the condition did not yield satisfactory results until the 1950s, when an immigrant orthopedic surgeon named **Ignacio Ponseti** (1914–2009) introduced a painless, non-invasive, low-cost procedure to correct clubfoot with a 95% success rate. Ponseti, born in Menorca, Spain in 1914, studied medicine at Barcelona University and served as a medic in the Orthopedic and Fracture Service during the Spanish Civil War. After immigrating to the US in 1941, he joined the orthopedic faculty at the University of Iowa, where he focused his research on congenital and childhood developmental bone and joint and skeletal growth disorders.

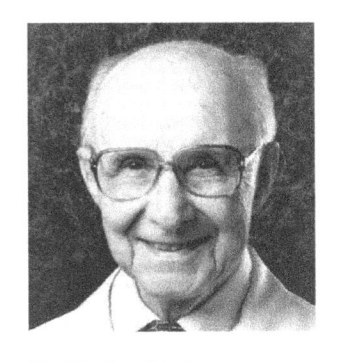

Fig 29. Spanish-American orthopedic surgeon Ignacio Ponseti who introduced a novel non-operative method for treating congenital clubfoot deformity that is being used worldwide. (Ponseti International)

Ponseti's most remarkable innovation was in the management of clubfoot deformity. He developed a groundbreaking, non-surgical treatment for the deformity, which became known worldwide as the Ponseti Method. This noninvasive procedure consists of manually stretching the soft tissues of the foot and ankle, followed by the application of a series of casts that gradually align the child's foot. This may require five serial casts and one to two months to give the child a new chance at a disability-free life without needing surgery. The Ponseti method **(Fig 29)** is now the gold standard treatment for clubfoot globally and endorsed by many international organizations, including the World Health Organization, National Institutes of Health, American Academy of Orthopedic Surgeons, Pediatric Orthopedic Society of North America, and European Pediatric Orthopedic Society. During the International Clubfoot Symposium of 2007, a report estimated that 10,000 children were successfully treated with the technique around the world.

The Ponseti International Association for the Advancement of Clubfoot Treatment was founded in 2006 to improve the treatment of children born with clubfeet through education, research, and improved access to care. World Clubfoot Day was announced in 2013 by the Ponseti International Association and is celebrated on June 3rd annually, commemorating Ponseti's birthday with the purpose of increasing awareness of the deformity and its prevention using the Ponseti method.

Cardiology and Immigrant Cardiologists

The field of cardiology traces its history back to 1628 when William Harvey, an English physician, published his observations on the heart and circulation, including congestive heart failure. In 1895, the Dutch physician Willem Einthoven invented the first practical electrocardiograph (EKG), for which he received the Nobel Prize in Physiology or Medicine in 1924. Other European and American physicians, including immigrant Americans, contributed to the field and improved upon the original EKG, leading to modern advances such as wearable devices that can record an EKG for less than $100.

One of the earliest immigrant physicians to emphasize the importance of preventing heart disease was **Isidore Snapper**, a Dutch-born internist who graduated from the University of Amsterdam in 1911. In 1938, he moved to New York and collaborated with the Rockefeller Foundation, conducting epidemiologic research on cardiovascular disease in China. Snapper's research found that plant-based diets, high in linoleic acid, lowered blood cholesterol levels, a cause of heart disease. While in China, Snapper was taken prisoner by the Japanese but was later exchanged for a Japanese diplomat captured in Indonesia. After his release, he continued to advocate for prevention in New York City and Chicago.

In the US, cardiology became a branch of internal medicine that deals with disorders of the heart and cardiovascular system. The specialty was established in the early 20th century by a group of physicians, led by **Franz Groedel** (1881–1951), a German-born physician who emigrated to the US in 1933. Groedel's focus shifted from cardiac radiology to clinical cardiology and electrocardiography, and he developed the concept of the unipolar chest lead or precordial electrode. Groedel's legacy is the American College of Cardiology, which he founded in 1949, and which is now a thriving professional society with 48 chapters in the US and Puerto Rico and over 54,000 members. The American Heart Association was founded in 1948 by cardiologist Paul White.

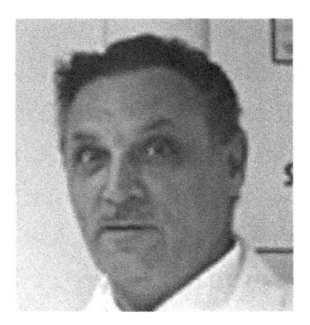

Fig 30. Immigrant cardiologist Eliot Corday contributed to development of continuous EKG recording, was ardent advocate for heart health and secured federal funding for cardiovascular research. (Cardiology magazine)

The Corday Prize, one of the most prestigious awards in the field of cardiology, was established in 2012 to recognize physicians and scientists whose groundbreaking research advances the practice of heart medicine. The prize was named after **Eliot Corday** (1897–1956), a Canadian-American cardiologist who played a crucial role in the development of continuous EKG recording in ambulatory patients and made radioisotope research that was a precursor to current nuclear cardiology. Corday **(Fig 30)** also received federal funding for the first international circuit course to Asian countries, which became a successful program known as the "Medical Peace Corps." Corday and philanthropist Mary Lasker united in support of funding for the National Institutes of Health, and Corday was invited by President Ronald Reagan to head the US Information Agency's Medical Science

Advisory Committee. Corday and cardiovascular surgeon Michael DeBakey successfully advocated before Congress for federal funding of cardiovascular research, leading to the passage of the Heart Disease, Cancer, and Stroke Amendments of 1965.

Karl Landsteiner and Erwin Popper (1879-1955) announced in Vienna that polio was caused by a virus after they injected monkeys with material prepared by grinding spinal cord tissue from children who had died from the disease. The first polio epidemic in the US occurred in Vermont in June of 1894, resulting in 18 deaths and 132 cases of permanent paralysis. In the summer of 1916, another polio epidemic broke out in the US, and more than 2000 people died in New York City alone. Between 1948 and 1955, several polio epidemics occurred in the US, causing around 16,000 cases of paralytic poliomyelitis each year on average. The development of vaccines by Salk and Sabin helped control the spread of the disease in industrialized countries worldwide.

On August 9th, 1921, Franklin D. Roosevelt, a practicing lawyer in New York City, fell into a cold lake while vacationing in Canada and contracted polio. Initially diagnosed with a "summer cold" by a physician, he was later diagnosed with a blood clot in the spinal cord by another physician. After paralysis set in, a third physician recommended that he consult with the Harvard Infantile Paralysis Commission. On August 20th, FDR contacted the Commission and spoke with **Samuel Levine** (1891–1966), a cardiologist and Polish immigrant based in Boston who was the first to diagnose him with acute poliomyelitis. Levine had graduated from Harvard Medical School in 1914 and acquired a reputation as an outstanding cardiologist at Brigham and Women's Hospital in Boston.

Levine was known for his innovative approach to treating heart attack patients, recommending that they be moved out of bed and into a chair just two days after their acute heart attack, contrary to conventional treatments that mandated several weeks of bed rest. Despite his warnings about the harmful effects of recumbency, it took years for the "armchair" treatment of heart attack patients to become widely accepted. Levine was also recruited by the Harvard Infantile Paralysis Commission to deal with the caseload of the 1916 poliomyelitis epidemic, where he acquired knowledge of the disease that led to his diagnosis of FDR five years later.

Levine was self-critical and warned his learners about iatrogenic disease caused by doctors. He was troubled by the prevalent polypharmacy, where patients are prescribed or take over-the-counter medications that can be more harmful than beneficial. The Levine Scale, Levine's Sign, and Lown-Ganong-Levine syndrome are all named after him. The Samuel Albert Levine Cardiac Unit at Brigham and Women's Hospital is also named in his honor. In 1954, New York investment banker Charles Merrell endowed the Samuel A. Levine Professorship at Harvard Medical School.

In 1929, a German physician named Werner Forssmann did something that had never been done before: he applied local anesthetic to his arm, inserted a catheter into his vein, and advanced it all the way to his heart, not knowing if the catheter might penetrate his vein or heart, which could have had dire consequences. The purpose of this successful self-experiment was to investigate the hypothesis and feasibility of delivering drugs or radioisotope dyes directly into the heart. Forssmann's work came to the attention of two cardiologists in the US, Dickinson Richards and an immigrant-Frenchman who applied Forssmann's method to heart disease patients, thus the cardiac catheterization technique was born. The immigrant-American cardiologist was **André Cournand** (1895-1988), and these three physicians won one of the highest awards for their achievements.

Cournand was born in Paris and received his early education in France. He obtained a bachelor's degree from the Sorbonne in 1913, and his medical education began in 1914 but was interrupted when he joined the army. He completed his medical education in 1925 and

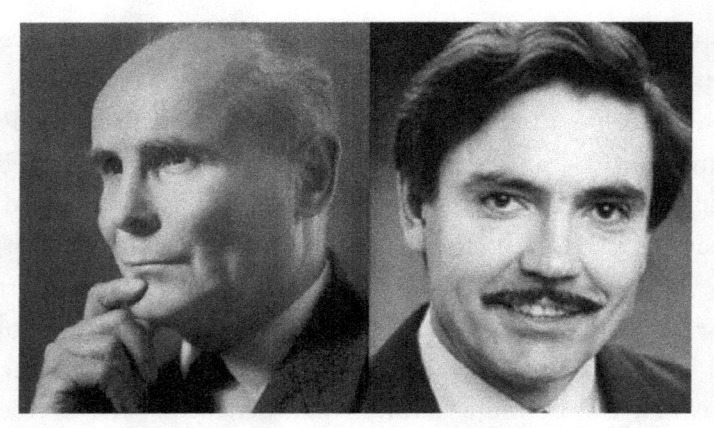

Fig 31. Immigrant cardiologists André Cournand (left) and Andreas Grüntzig (right) who developed and popularized cardiac catheterization by Cournand and balloon angioplasty by Grüntzig. (PCR online and Wikipedia)

earned his MD degree from the Faculté de Médecine de Paris in 1930. He emigrated to the US in 1930 and secured a residency in internal medicine at Columbia University Division at Bellevue Hospital, NY. In 1941, he became a naturalized US citizen. Cournand **(Fig 31)** became a professor at Columbia University College of Physicians and Surgeons and worked in the Chest Service of Bellevue Hospital, where he conducted his research and clinical work. He became internationally renowned for revolutionizing cardiology and pulmonology with his groundbreaking research.

Cournand's most important innovation was accomplished in collaboration with the other physicians, which revolutionized heart disease diagnosis and treatment. In 1956, along with Forssmann and Richards, Cournand was awarded the Nobel Prize in Physiology or Medicine for the development of cardiac catheterization. The technique involves safely threading a thin, flexible tube through a vein to reach the heart, which has made it possible today to diagnose and treat heart conditions such as clogged arteries (thrombosis) and irregular heartbeats (arrhythmia) early on. Cardiac catheterization was the precursor to today's interventional cardiology practice.

In 1961, a Lithuanian-immigrant cardiologist made one of the most important life-saving techniques in the US using a device that has saved millions of heart disease patients since then. Yet, this man did not receive the Nobel Prize that he deserved for his revolutionary work; rather, fortune favored this man by winning the Nobel Peace Prize for another accomplishment: social activism. The man was **Bernard Lown** (1921-2021), who was born in Utena, Lithuania and emigrated with his family to Maine when he was 14. He studied zoology at the University of Maine, and in 1945 earned an MD from Johns Hopkins University School of Medicine. He completed cardiology training at Brigham and Women's Hospital in Boston, where Samuel Levine was his mentor and later collaborator. Both Lown and Levine realized that the high mortality of heart attack patients was most likely due to a strict regimen of long bed rest that led to complications such as pulmonary embolism, which led to the adoption of chair treatment by the medical community.

In 1775, a Danish veterinarian named Peter Abildgaard conducted an experiment on a hen in which he applied an electric shock to its head, causing it to become unconscious. He then administered a second shock to the chest, which revived the hen. He repeated the experiment, which resulted in the chicken being stunned and walking erratically. However, the hen recovered the following day and even laid an egg. In 1899, Swiss physiologists Jean Prevost and Frederic Batelli induced ventricular fibrillation in a dog using low-voltage electric shocks and reversed the condition with higher charges. Lown learned of these experiments and raised awareness about sudden cardiac death, highlighting that it is survivable and reversible, and that patients can be resuscitated successfully. Until the 1950s, ventricular fibrillation, a leading cause of cardiac arrest, was treated with alternating current electric shock derived from a wall socket. In 1959, Lown demonstrated through animal research that alternating current could burn the heart muscle, and that it could be lethal, causing ventricular fibrillation. In 1961, he and his colleagues proved that a specific direct current (DC) waveform could reverse ventricular fibrillation, restore a normal heart rhythm, and avoid injuring the heart or chest skeletal muscles. Lown used his defibrillator invention to treat tachycardia by preventing ventricular fibrillation through a method called "Cardioversion."

The defibrillator became invaluable during heart surgery, restoring cardiac beat after major heart operations. Lown's DC defibrillator and cardioverter improved the survival of patients with coronary heart disease worldwide and advanced modern cardiac surgery. Portable defibrillators are now used outside hospitals, carried by ambulances and even installed in restrooms in some European countries. Lown's defibrillator use was further evolved by the invention of the implantable device, known as the implantable cardioverter-defibrillator.

Digitalis toxicity was a major cause of fatality among patients with congestive heart failure receiving the drug. Lown discovered the critical role of potassium in the safe use of digitalis. As a result of his research, long-acting digitalis use was abandoned in favor of short-acting, and he advocated the use of the anesthetic lidocaine as a drug treatment for controlling heartbeat disturbances.

In early 1961, Lown **(Fig 32)** began his social activism by calling on a group of physicians from Boston to address the threat of nuclear war between the USSR and the US, resulting in the establishment of a new organization called Physicians for Social Responsibility. In 1980, with the help of physicians and first-year Harvard medical students, he formed the International Physicians for the Prevention of Nuclear War (IPPNW). By 1985, this organization was represented by 135,000 physicians in 60 countries. That same year, Lown and Eugene Chazov accepted the 1985 Nobel Peace Prize on behalf of IPPNW. Lown received numerous awards, including having a bridge connecting the cities of Lewiston and Auburn in Maine renamed The Bernard Lown Peace Bridge. Other honors include the Bernard Lown Educational Award at the Brigham and Women's Hospital and the Lown Scholars Program at the Harvard School of Public Health. Lown also wrote a book, *The Lost*

Art of Healing (1999), about the importance of practicing compassion towards patients, and linking science to the art and skill of medicine to improve doctor-patient relationships.

Coronary atherosclerosis or arteriosclerosis is a heart condition where plaque forms on the walls of arteries, which can lead to narrowing of the lumen. The primary risk factor for this condition is an elevated level of abnormal cholesterol in the blood. Severe constriction of the arteries can cause symptoms of angina, and if the plaque ruptures, vessel occlusion may occur, leading to a myocardial infarction or heart attack. Coronary artery disease is the leading cause of death and disability in the developed world. While major heart bypass surgery is an option, non-operative treatment of angina can prevent the onset of a heart attack. One of the most common noninvasive procedures for the treatment of coronary artery disease is balloon angioplasty, a technique that was first used by German-American cardiologist **Andreas Grüntzig** (1939-1985) to expand the lumens of narrowed arteries. Grüntzig was born in Dresden just before WWII and grew up in Leipzig, where he received an early education. He began his medical studies at Heidelberg University in 1958, graduated six years later, and joined the same university's Institute for Social and Occupational Medicine, investigating risk factors for cardiovascular disease.

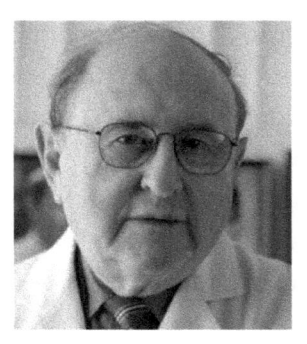

Fig 32. Immigrant cardiologist Bernard Lown devised the defibrillator for cardioversion to treat tachycardia and ventricular fibrillation. His social activism won him a Nobel Prize. (Maine Public)

American radiologist Charles Dotter invented angioplasty and the catheter-delivered stent and first used it to treat diseased arteries in the limbs. In the 1960s, Grüntzig attended a lecture by Dotter in Frankfort, where he learned the technique and investigated its application to the heart. In 1977, using a catheter he built in his kitchen, Grüntzig **(Fig 31)** performed the first successful coronary angioplasty on a wide-awake patient who remained angina-free for at least ten years. That same year, Grüntzig presented the results of four angioplasty cases at the American Heart Association meeting, which led to the adoption of the technique in the US. Grüntzig spent the remainder of his career at Emory University in Atlanta, focusing his research on angiology and epidemiology, and teaching others the proper technique to ensure good outcomes. By the 1990s, the angioplasty technique was used more frequently than coronary artery bypass surgery to treat lumen stenosis of the coronary arteries.

Ironically, Grüntzig developed coronary artery disease and had a balloon angioplasty in 1985, and he went back to work the same day. Later that year, while flying an airplane, his plane crashed, and he died in Forsyth, Georgia.

Ultrasound and Immigrant Ultrasound Physicians

Medical ultrasound has undergone an evolutionary process to become the technology we know today. In 1877, brothers Jacques and Pierre Curie discovered the piezoelectric effect, which is the ability of certain materials to generate an electric charge in response to mechanical stress. After the sinking of the Titanic, French physicist Paul Langevin, a student of Pierre Curie and later a lover of widowed Marie Curie, was commissioned in 1915 to create a device to detect objects on the ocean floor in the hopes of locating the Titanic. Langevin invented a hydrophone, which did not find the Titanic, but helped him develop the technique of ultrasonic submarine detection.

Medical ultrasound is often used to image the human body for disease diagnosis by generating high-frequency sound waves that are beyond the range of human hearing. An ultrasound probe transmits high-pitched pulses that are reflected from a hidden organ and create an image called a sonogram. Scottish physician Ian Donald used ultrasound to examine a woman with a large pelvic tumor in 1952 and diagnosed an ovarian cyst. Two years later, he scanned the head of a fetus in-utero. Ultrasound scanners were put into commercial use in the 1960s, and obstetricians quickly utilized and heavily relied on them to measure fetal head circumference and maternal pelvic outlet to determine the feasibility of vaginal delivery; ultrasound can also be used to detect fetal deformities. Medical ultrasound can identify cysts, tumors, and the integrity of muscles and tendons. Doppler ultrasound determines blood flow in arteries to detect any blockages, whereas a heart echocardiogram produces a heart image and evaluates its function. The most common use of high-frequency ultrasound as a therapeutic modality is performing lithotripsy, which is a noninvasive procedure that generates shock waves to destroy kidney and gallbladder stones. Ultrasound can also be used to generate deep heat for physical therapy and other interventions.

In 1942, **Karl Dussik** (1908-1968), an Austrian-born immigrant physician, was the first to use medical ultrasound by transmitting an ultrasonic beam through a patient's skull to detect a brain tumor. Dussik began his professional career as a dentist, but later graduated from the University of Vienna Medical School in 1931 and practiced as a neurologist and psychiatrist. Having learned that ultrasonic waves had been employed in detecting submarines and schools of fish, he began exploring the use of ultrasonics in medical diagnosis in 1937. He soon became the first to use ultrasound as a diagnostic method in human subjects, a procedure which he named "Hyperphonography." In 1941, he published his idea of using ultrasound as a diagnostic device. In 1947, Dussik developed an apparatus to make images of the brain and its ventricles by recording the echoes of the ultrasonic transmissions using the piezoelectric effect. One year later, he and Wolf-Dieter Keidel were the only two investigators to present on the use of ultrasound in medical diagnostics at The First Congress of Ultrasound in Medicine in Germany.

Dussik emigrated to the US with his wife and two children in 1951, where he took up an appointment at Boston State Hospital. Shortly thereafter, he published his experience with 300 cases of ultrasound investigation of brain pathologies. With funding from the National Institute of Health, he shifted his research to therapeutic ultrasound and its energy distribution in the treatment of arthritis and multiple sclerosis. He also explored ultrasound use in physical therapy.

In 1954, Dussik joined the executive committee of The American Institute of Ultrasound in Medicine, and in 1956, he attended a historical conference in Bioacoustics hosted by MIT, where he met Swedish-American neurosurgeon **Petter Lindström** and British-American physician **John Wild**, both immigrants like him. Dussik's pioneering work in ultrasound had inspired others, such as Oklahoma-born neurosurgeon Thomas Ballantine Jr., to explore its potential for diagnosing intracranial lesions. In 1958, Dussik published his last paper, which was the first on measuring articular tissue with ultrasound. Afterward, he served as the Assistant to the Commissioner of Mental Health of the Commonwealth of Massachusetts until his death.

Meanwhile, researchers in Europe were also experimenting with ultrasound. In 1953, Swedish physician Inge Elder and German physicist C. Hellmuth Hertz performed the first echocardiogram. Scottish engineer Tom Brown patented the technology in 1957 and collaborated with English obstetrician Ian Donald and British physician John MacVicar to develop an ultrasound scanner that could capture images of the human body. In 1964, Donald used an ultrasound machine to observe fetal echoes in the uterus and monitor fetal development during pregnancy.

In 1946, a physician from England emigrated to the US and, by 1951, he and his team had developed a noninvasive way to detect breast cancer and other tumors using ultrasound scans that reflected onto a fluorescent television screen. **John Wild** (1914-2009), born in Kent and raised in London, became a doctor in 1942 and served in the Royal Army Medical Corps during WWII. Afterward, he joined the general surgery department at the University of Minnesota, where he pursued research on using high-frequency ultrasound to detect injuries of the intestines. Wild's team gained access to better equipment in 1951, which allowed them to distinguish between healthy and cancerous tissue in abdominal organs and breast tissue. In the same year, Wild published his innovation in *The Lancet*, followed by *Science* in 1952. He and his team were the first to design equipment specifically for scanning breast tissue and differentiating between cystic and solid masses using ultrasonography.

Breast ultrasound continues to be used today—alongside mammography—to diagnose breast cancer and other tumors. While ultrasound uses high-frequency sound waves to create an image of the breast without any radiation, mammography uses low-dose radiation to obtain breast images. Although mammography is widely used today as the primary diagnostic tool for detecting breast tumors, ultrasound can be a useful adjunct to mammography. Although Dussik was the first physician to use ultrasound to visualize the brain, his first images were blurred because of artifacts produced by the equipment and were not clinically relevant. Wild's work in ultrasonography, on the other hand, produced some of the first practical and reliable higher resolution images. In recognition of his innovations in the field of ultrasound imaging, Wild was honored in 1991 with the Japan Prize, which included a cash award of 10 million yen ($370,000). Although others had contributed to the field before him, Wild is considered by some to be the "father of medical ultrasound."

Psychiatry and Immigrant Psychiatrists

In the 4th century BCE, Hippocrates theorized that mental disorders had physiological roots. In ancient times, religious leaders resorted to exorcism to treat mental disorders, often using barbaric methods such as drilling holes in the skull to release demons. In the early 9th century, Baghdad was the first city to build "dar-al-shifa" (houses of cure), which later spread throughout Arab countries. These early hospitals contained wards for mentally ill patients. Medieval Islamic physicians including Rhazes and Avicenna also wrote about mental disorders.

Johann Weyer (1515-1588), a Dutch physician who lived in the 16th century, wrote against the persecution of witches during a time when they were often tortured and burned at the stake by Christian authorities. In his book "De Praestigiis Daemonum et Incantationibus ac Venificiis" (On the Illusions of the Demons and on Spells and Poisons) published in 1563, he emphasized the importance of consulting a physician after women were accused of witchcraft. Although he did not deny the existence of the devil, he was the first to use the term "mentally ill" for some women accused of witchcraft. Some science historians consider Weyer the father of psychiatry, and his book was banned by the Catholic Church.

Specialized institutions were built in medieval Europe to house people with mental disorders but did not provide them with treatments. In 13th century Europe, patients with mental problems were isolated from the rest of the community and locked up in facilities with deplorable conditions. Bethlem Royal Hospital in London is one of the oldest lunatic asylums; it was founded in 1247, during the reign of Henry III, not as a hospital but as a religious house for the insane. Although around 1330 it was designated as a hospital, it continued using mechanical restraints and solitary confinements for the insane. In the 17th century, at Bethlem Hospital, those deemed dangerous continued to be chained or locked in isolated quarters. Many privately run asylums for the insane proliferated in Europe, but their treatment was far from humane and no less cruel and barbaric.

French physician Philippe Pinel's book *Treatise on Insanity* (1801) shed light on the horrifying treatment of the mentally ill in French asylums. He advocated for a more humane approach to treatment, arguing that the mentally ill should be treated with kindness instead of brutal methods such as bleeding, beating, chaining, starvation, and forced vomiting. Pinel's compassionate method led to a decrease in mortality rates and improvements in the condition of many patients, earning him recognition as a founder of the psychiatry specialty. Despite his influential work, some doctors continued to use inhumane methods to treat the mentally ill, such as Benjamin Rush's infamous chair, which restrained patients for days on end.

In the 18th century, attitudes towards the mentally ill began to shift towards benevolent treatment. By the beginning of the 19th century, psychiatry had made advances in the diagnosis of mental illness and ushered in the modern era of providing care for the mentally ill. Sigmund Freud, an Austrian psychiatrist, introduced the clinical method of psychoanalysis for evaluating and treating the pathology of the psyche through dialogue between the patient and a psychoanalyst in his book *Interpretation of Dreams* (1899). His work had a significant impact on psychiatrists of his time and those who followed. The integration of psychoanalysis and general psychiatry gave rise to dynamic psychiatry and psychotherapy.

In the 1800s, physicians began to recognize that certain areas of the brain were responsible for specific functions, leading to the belief that brain surgery targeting specific areas may cure mental illness. Lobotomy, the severance of connections to and from the frontal cortex responsible for personality, became popular in the 1900s. The process involved drilling holes in the skull and using a sharp instrument to cut into the brain tissue. Lobotomy was used to "cure" various mental disorders, including schizophrenia and depression. American physician Walter Freeman popularized psychosurgery in the mid-1940s and performed transorbital frontal lobotomies, which involved placing an ice pick as an instrument into the eye socket below the upper eyelid, hammering the pick into the brain, and swiveling it from side to side to mangle brain tissue. Patients who underwent this mutilating procedure experienced devastating complications such as brain hemorrhage, abscess, and permanent emotional dullness, epilepsy, dementia, and even death. Freeman performed 3,400 lobotomies during his nationwide tours. Between 1936 and 1956, approximately 60,000 such procedures were performed in the US. President Kennedy's sister Rosemary was subjected to a lobotomy at age 23 by her father, Freeman, and James Watts, with the promise to make her happy and content. The procedure left her with the mental capacity of a toddler, paralysis, urinary incontinence, and incoherence, and she was institutionalized for the rest of her life.

Despite widespread criticism and warnings from the AMA about the procedure, Freeman continued to perform countless lobotomies until he was banned from operating in 1967 after one of his patients died from a brain hemorrhage following a third lobotomy. Due to ethical concerns, lobotomy was nearly abandoned. The procedure was portrayed in the movie *One Flew Over the Cuckoo's Nest* (1975), which won five Academy Awards, and in the biopic *Frances* (1982), which depicted the complications of involuntary lobotomy.

Electro-convulsive Therapy (ECT) is another treatment modality based on the idea that inducing a seizure may improve mental illness. Italian physicians first used a crude technique of ECT, which was introduced to North America in the 1940s for the treatment of severe depression and acute attacks of schizophrenia. However, post-procedure, treated patients encountered aphasia, cognitive blunting, and a long recovery time. In 1944, Russian-born physician **Wladimir Liberson** (1904-1994) refined the technique and made it more practical. Despite not being a psychiatrist, Liberson made important contributions to the field of psychiatry. He was born in Russia, received his medical degree from the University of Paris in 1936, came to the US in 1940, and earned a Ph.D. in physiology at the University of Montreal in 1951. He focused on rehabilitation medicine and conducted research in neurophysiology and clinical work at hospitals in Hartford, Chicago, Miami, and New York in Brooklyn-Cumberland Medical Center. His research resulted in making ECT safer, more tolerable, and with fewer side effects.

Liberson's research extended to electromyography, which measures muscular electrical activity, electroencephalograms, which record the spontaneous electrical activity of the brain, and evoked potentials, which is a method in which a computer analyzes brain waves. He was instrumental in establishing the American Electroencephalography Society, served as its president, and became the president of both the American Rehabilitation and Clinical Evoked Potential societies. Liberson died in Miami. The 1960s and 70s witnessed an explosion of research in neurophysiology and neurochemistry, and ECT is now seldom used; behavioral therapy and medications have become more popular.

A psychiatrist is a physician who, after obtaining a medical degree, seeks residency training for the diagnosis, prevention, and treatment of patients with mental disorders. Today, the field of psychiatry has expanded immensely with many subspecialties that require additional fellowship training. Unlike psychiatry, which is a medical specialty, psychology is an academic discipline that is also vast in scope, crossing the boundaries between the natural and social sciences. Psychologists are social scientists who aim to understand the behavior and cognition of individuals and groups by conducting research on perception, attention, emotion, intelligence, experience, motivation, brain functioning, and personality. However, psychologists have also been tasked with advising and sometimes participating in the enhanced interrogation techniques at black sites.

Next, we will look at the stories of three immigrant men born in the 19th century, who became physicians and psychiatrists, emigrated to the US, and made important advancements in their field.

Victor of Aveyron was a French feral child who grew up in the woods of southern France, isolated from society, and was found at the age of nine. He became known as "The Wild Boy of Aveyron." The child was deemed mentally retarded, and at the time, mentally retarded people were regarded as untreatable and were isolated from society. However, the French physician Jean Itard believed otherwise. He dedicated years of his career to teaching the feral child to communicate and contended that the boy's mental deficiency was due to a lack of human interaction. A young physician who later became an American citizen was inspired by Itard's accomplishment, trained with him, and became a psychiatrist also teaching mentally retarded children. This young physician was **Édouard Séguin** (1812-1880), who was born in the small town of Clamecy in central France. While studying and working in Paris under Itard, an educator of the deaf-mute, Itard encouraged Seguin to pursue a career in psychiatry treating mentally challenged children. In 1840, Seguin established the first private school in Paris for educating people with intellectual disabilities and published in French *The Moral Treatment, Hygiene, and Education of Idiots and Other Backward Children* (1846), which was the earliest textbook addressing the special needs of children with intellectual disabilities.

In 1848, Séguin emigrated to the US and settled in New York. He received his MD from the University of the City of New York in 1861 and later established several schools in various cities for the treatment of the mentally handicapped. In 1866, he published "Idiocy: and its Treatment by the Physiological Method." In his schools, Séguin stressed the importance of developing self-reliance and independence for the mentally disabled by giving them a combination of physical and intellectual tasks. He believed that patients with mental retardation who were labeled as "idiots" could be trained to perform tasks and learn. He spent much time focusing on their vocational training and self-care skills.

Séguin recognized the potential benefits of the physiological method of treating handicapped children and believed that mental deficiency was caused by a nervous system disorder that could be cured through a process of motor and sensory training. He also devised a special "physiological thermometer" and described a medical "Séguin's signal" where involuntary muscle contraction occurs before an epileptic attack. He became the first president of the American Association on Mental Retardation. Séguin is considered the first great teacher in the field of disabilities and is remembered for his work with children having cognitive impairments.

The US has one of the highest rates of incarceration among Western societies, and prison inmates have a significantly high prevalence of psychiatric disorders. In the US, inmates are the only group that has a constitutionally recognized right to healthcare, including mental illnesses. Correctional psychiatry evolved as a sub-subspecialty from the need to provide treatment to many delinquents behind bars with mental illness. One of the earliest advocates of engaging psychiatrists in prisons was **Adolf Meyer** (1866-1950), an immigrant psychiatrist. Meyer was born in Niererwenningen, Switzerland, and received his MD from the University of Zurich in 1892. He studied neurology abroad under renowned physicians, including the French Jean-Martin Charcot, who described several diseases named after him, most notably Charcot-Marie-Tooth disease. This is a form of genetic muscular atrophy where the patient develops progressive weakness and muscle paralysis of the hands and feet. The work of Charcot with hypnosis and hysteria influenced Meyer to study psychiatry and focus on neuroanatomy and neurophysiology.

Meyer emigrated to the US in 1892 and was influenced by the pragmatist philosophers William James and John Dewey. He first practiced and taught neurology at the University of Chicago, and later in Worcester, Massachusetts, all while publishing research in neuropathology and psychiatry. After being appointed as director of the Pathological Institute of the New York State Hospital system in 1902, which later became The Psychiatric Institute, he imported Sigmund Freud's ideas and shaped much of American psychiatry. Meyer became Professor of Psychiatry at Cornell University in 1904, but ultimately settled at Johns Hopkins Hospital where he founded the Henry Phipps Psychiatric Clinic in 1913, which became a research center and a renowned mental institute. Meyer introduced a novel model of patient care combining clinical and laboratory elements.

Meyer was one of the most influential psychiatrists of the early 20th century, popularizing his discipline and making seminal contributions by introducing his ideas to the field of psychobiology. He served as president of the American Psychiatric Association and on the advisory council of the American Eugenics Society, but he contradicted the genetic determinism that fostered scientific racism in the first half of the 20th century. He was a strong advocate of engaging psychiatrists in prisons, schools, and other community venues.

While serving as Professor of Psychiatry at Johns Hopkins School of Medicine, Meyer influenced several of his aspiring students, some of whom became accomplished psychiatrists, making substantial contributions to American psychiatry. Two of these were immigrants: the Austrian-born **Abraham Brill** and the Scottish-born **Charles Campbell**. **Leo Kanner**, an Austrian-born psychiatrist, founded the first child psychiatry clinic in the US at Johns Hopkins Hospital under Meyer's direction. Kanner is best known for his original work on autism.

During the summer of 1954, four teenagers who belonged to Brooklyn's Jewish community roamed the streets of Brooklyn, assaulting girls, beating up and torturing homeless people, and ultimately killed two men: one by drowning and the other by beating. Robert Trachtenberg was 15, Melvin Mittman, and Jerome Lieberman were 17, and Jack Koslow was 18. After their arrest, two of the boys bragged about the murders and referred to the homeless as "social parasites." The murders committed by these boys became a cause célèbre, attracting national media frenzy. Koslow admitted that he read comic books before the murders and saw himself as a crime-fighting hero. Koslow and Mittman were eventually found guilty of felony murder.

During the trial of the "Brooklyn Thrill Killers," a psychiatrist named **Fredric Wertham** (1895-1981) was appointed by the court to provide his expertise. He concluded that comic books were responsible for juvenile delinquency and cited the boys as an example of the potential harm caused by these books. Wertham was a German-immigrant physician born in Nuremberg to a Jewish family. He studied at King's College London, graduated with an MD from the University of Würzburg in Germany in 1921, and became a psychiatrist after visiting Sigmund Freud. In 1922, he emigrated to the US and worked in the Phipps Psychiatric Clinic at Johns Hopkins Hospital.

In 1932, Wertham accepted a senior staff position at the Bellevue Mental Hygiene Clinic and conducted forensic psychiatric examinations of convicted felons that were used in courts. He also opened the Lafargue Clinic in Harlem in 1946, which was a low-cost psychiatric facility financed by contributions for treating poor black teenagers. Wertham was concerned with the adverse effects of violent images in mass media and the influence of comic books on children's development. In his book "Seduction of the Innocent" (1954), he claimed that comic books with violent titles caused youth to become criminals. Wertham also testified before Congress in 1954 and wrote articles on comic books and their promotion. The outrage surrounding the "Brooklyn Thrill Killers" case fueled the public backlash against comic books, leading to the creation of the Comics Code Authority in 1954.

After Wertham's involvement in the trial, some comic book series were banned by the State of NY, and the Supreme Court of the US upheld the ban in its *Kingsley Books, Inc. v. Brown* 1957 ruling. Wertham's writings about racial segregation were also used as evidence in the landmark *Supreme Court case Brown v. Board of Education*. Wertham wrote several books dealing with violence, murder, euthanasia, and mental illness and was associated with a group of left-wing intellectuals, mostly German immigrants, who argued that mass culture was a destructive force in society. Before retirement, Wertham became a professor of psychiatry at New York University. The story of Fredric Wertham and comic books in the 1940s and 1950s is detailed in the documentary "Diagram for Delinquents" (2014).

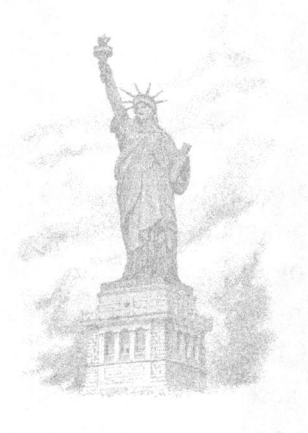

CHAPTER 9

Award-Winning Physicians

Awards and prizes are an important way to honor the contribution of individuals or organizations in recognition of their excellence in many fields. Such distinctions are common in every industry, from the Arts to business to sports. Awards ceremonies such as the Oscars or the Olympics punctuate and underpin our conception of human achievement. In no field is this less evident than in the natural and social sciences.

More than 150 major awards are bestowed globally in the field of Medicine. Canada and Europe offer many of these prizes, but the majority of these are offered by US institutions. Awarding bodies include major medical organizations and foundations, universities, and philanthropists. They offer opportunities to sponsor individuals who have made a significant contribution to enhancing diagnosis, treatment, and prevention of disease.

Three of the oldest and most distinguished of these awards are the Nobel Prize, the Pulitzer Prize, and the Lasker Awards. The Nobel Prize recognizes contributions to society; the Pulitzer Prize honors literary achievements; meanwhile, the Lasker is offered for excellence in various branches of the medical field. Two of the founders of these three awards were immigrants.

Nobel Prize

Alfred Bernhard Nobel (1833 – 1896) was a Swedish businessman, chemist, engineer, inventor, and philanthropist. He attended school in Stockholm and excelled in chemistry and languages including English, French, German, and Russian. Nobel came to the US to study under **John Ericsson** (1803 –1889) a Swedish-American and inventor of the steam locomotive.

Nobel experimented with the controlled, commercial use of nitroglycerin as an explosive. His invention of dynamite began by mixing nitroglycerine with gunpowder, which he called 'blasting oil.' His intention was to help with the construction of roads, railways, bridges, ports, and towns. In 1864, Emil—Alfred's brother—was producing this oil when an unexpected blast killed five people, including Emil. In 1867, Alfred would later make nitroglycerine safer to ignite by mixing it with sand and inventing a detonator—the blasting cap—which would become known as 'dynamite' and for which he would be dubbed 'the Merchant of Death.'

In 1888, one newspaper would report that the 'King of Dynamite,' Alfred Nobel had died of a heart attack. No one was more shocked to read his obituary, than Alfred himself: the paper had in fact erroneously reported the death of his brother, Ludvig, as his own. By the time of his actual death, however, he had become one of the wealthiest men in Europe. Appalled by the use of his most famous invention in the development of military weaponry, he had decided to leave a very different legacy. Nobel willed his entire estate to the creation of a set of annual prizes awarded to those who had contributed great service to mankind.

The Nobel Prize was established posthumously in 1901 and consists of a set of awards given annually by Swedish and Norwegian institutions in six categories, including Chemistry, Literature, Peace, Physics, Physiology/Medicine, and Economics. These prizes are widely regarded as the most prestigious awards in the world. Since its inception until 2022, the Nobel Prizes have been awarded 615 times to 989 people and organizations from around the world. Many of the winners have been immigrant-Americans whose outstanding scientific and research accomplishments have brought honor to the US. In recent decades, an increasing number of Nobel Prize winners in Physics, Medicine, and Chemistry have been immigrants to the US.

Immigrants to the US have comprised a significant share (15%) of all Nobel Laureates awarded from 1901 to 2022, with 148 individuals making contributions in various fields. In 2016, all six American winners of the Nobel Prize in economics and scientific fields were foreign-born. In 2017, eight of the Nobel Prize winners were Americans, two of whom were immigrants. Although there were no immigrant Nobel winners in 2018, in 2019, out of the 15 Nobel winners, 8 were Americans, and 5 of them were immigrants. Seven out of the 13 Nobel Prize winners in 2021 were from the US, and five of them were not born in America.

According to research from the National Foundation for American Policy, between 1901 and 1959, immigrants won 25 Nobel Prizes in Chemistry, Medicine, and Physics, but this number increased to 79 prizes between 1960 and 2016. Furthermore, from 2000 to 2017, immigrants were awarded 40 percent, or 31 out of 78, of the Nobel Prizes won by Americans in Chemistry, Medicine, and Physics.

Immigrant Physician Nobel Laureates

Physician scientists dedicate a significant amount of time to research and often make novel discoveries that enhance patient care and the field of medicine. The following are eight immigrant physician scientists who were recipients of the Nobel Prize.

The Belgian-American **Albert Claude** was mentioned earlier. After graduating from medical school, he worked at the Kaiser Wilhelm Institute for Biology in Germany and received a fellowship from the Belgian-American Educational Foundation for research in the US. Claude joined the Rockefeller Institute in New York, where he made his most pioneering accomplishment in cell biology by developing a cell fractionation technique that allowed him to explore the small universe of cells. In collaboration with colleagues, Claude used the electron microscope for the first time in the field of biology and identified components of cell organelles. Claude's pioneering work earned him the Louisa Gross Horwitz Prize. Together with two other immigrant physicians, **George Palade** and the Canadian-American cell biologist **Keith Porter**, Claude won the Paul Ehrlich and Ludwig Darmstaedter Prize. Lastly, he won the Nobel Prize in Physiology or Medicine in 1974 with his student George Palade and Christian de Duve.

George Palade (1912–2008) was born in Iași, Romania, and received his medical degree in 1940 from the Carol Davila School of Medicine in Bucharest, where he later became a faculty member. In 1946, he went to the US and engaged in research at the Biology Laboratory of New York University. He later joined Albert Claude at the Rockefeller Institute and became a US citizen in 1952. He accepted a position as a professor and the first Chairman of the Department of Cell Biology at Yale University Medical School, a professor at the University of California, San Diego in the Department of Cellular and Molecular Medicine, and later a Dean for Scientific Affairs in the School of Medicine at La Jolla, California.

Palade conducted research in cell biology and electron microscopy, focusing on the internal organization of cell structures such as ribosomes, mitochondria, chloroplasts, and Golgi apparatus. His groundbreaking discovery was made using a pulse-chase analysis experimental strategy, which confirmed the existence of a secretory pathway and the functional relationship between the Rough Endoplasmic Reticulum and the Golgi apparatus.

In recognition of his contributions, Palade was awarded the Louisa Gross Horwitz Prize from Columbia University in 1970, along with the Italian-American Nobel laureate **Renato Dulbecco**. He also received the Nobel Prize in Physiology and Medicine in 1974, which he shared with Albert Claude and Christian de Duve. Palade's cell fractionation process was developed in collaboration with Argentine-American physician and cell biologist **David Sabatini**. Additionally, Palade was elected as an honorary member of the American-Romanian Academy of Arts and Sciences, received the Golden Plate Award of the American Academy of Achievement, and became a founding member of the World Cultural Council and founding editor of the Annual Review of Cell and Developmental Biology.

Acetylcholine is an organic chemical that is found in the bodies of animals and humans, and it plays important roles in the central and peripheral nervous systems. In the cerebral cortex and hippocampus of the brain, it supports cognitive functions such as learning and memory. In the peripheral nerves, acetylcholine activates skeletal muscles, causing them to contract, and it is a major neurotransmitter in the autonomic nervous system. While it also has an influence on the sympathetic system, stimulating the body's fight or flight response, its more significant function in the parasympathetic system is to stimulate "rest-and-digest" or "feed and breed" activities that occur when a person is at rest, especially after eating, sexual arousal, salivation, lacrimation, urination, digestion, and defecation.

The existence of acetylcholine was unknown until 1921 when it was discovered by the immigrant physician scientist **Otto Loewi** (1873-1961). Loewi was born in Frankfurt, Germany and studied medicine at the University of Strasbourg. He worked at Goethe University and City Hospital in Frankfurt before focusing his work on pharmacology due to the high mortality rate from infectious disease. At the University of Marburg, he conducted research on metabolism, particularly protein synthesis. During his time at the University of Graz in Austria, he proved that animals could rebuild their body proteins from the degradation products, the amino acids, which was an important discovery for nutrition. Loewi also investigated how vital organs respond to chemical and electrical stimulation and established their dependence on epinephrine for adequate function. In his famous experiment on frogs in 1921, Loewi discovered how chemical messengers transmit nerve impulses, and the first chemical neurotransmitter he identified was acetylcholine. His experiment was the first to demonstrate that the endogenous release of a chemical substance could cause a response in the absence of electrical stimulation.

As a result of his pioneering work, Loewi was awarded the Nobel Prize in Physiology or Medicine in 1936, which he shared with British pharmacologist Sir Henry Dale. After Germany invaded Austria, Loewi moved to the United States in 1940, where he became a research professor at the New York University College of Medicine and later became a naturalized citizen in 1946.

Loewi observed that the removal of the pancreas from dogs, which created experimental diabetes, resulted in a change in the response of the eye to adrenaline. While this had no effect on normal dogs, dogs without a pancreas exhibited dilated pupils when adrenaline drops were applied to the eye. Based on Loewi's observation, physicians used this as a diagnostic test for acute pancreatitis.

Myasthenia gravis is an autoimmune disease characterized by muscle weakness and fatigue, commonly affecting the muscles of the eyes, face, swallowing, and walking. It is now known that the disease is caused by the body producing antibodies against acetylcholine receptors, which inhibits proper acetylcholine signal transmission. The condition can be treated with medications known as acetylcholinesterase inhibitors, and in some cases, by the surgical removal of the thymus gland in the upper chest area if a tumor is causing the problem.

Loewi received honorary doctorates from New York, Yale, Graz, and Frankfurt universities. He received many other awards from Bologna, Austria, Edinburg, England, and Germany.

Living organisms conduct thousands of chemical reactions that occur within cells. For cells to function normally, they may require a large amount of energy. Enzymes play an important catalytic role in the chemical processes required for the normal function of cells. Without enzymes, it would be impossible for cells to produce the large amount of energy needed under normal conditions. Most enzymes are proteins. There are 1300 enzymes identified in human cells, which fall into three categories: amylase, which breaks down starches and carbohydrates into sugars; protease, which breaks down proteins into amino acids; and lipase, which breaks down lipids, or fats and oils, into glycerol and fatty acids.

For enzymes to function, they need catalysts or coenzymes, which are non-protein chemical compounds or helper molecules that increase the rate of chemical reactions. A coenzyme binds to a protein molecule, forming an active enzyme. Some vitamins function as coenzymes; for example, the B group of vitamins serve as coenzymes necessary for enzymes involved in the formation of fats, carbohydrates, and proteins. Vitamin K is a coenzyme for blood coagulation. The iron (Fe) found in red blood cells allows hemoglobin to bind and release oxygen in the lungs and tissues during respiration.

Coenzyme A is necessary for various metabolic cycles, such as the synthesis and oxidation of fatty acids, which are essential for the structure of cell membranes. It was recently commercially produced by extraction from yeast. This enzyme was discovered by **Fritz Lipmann** (1899–1986), an immigrant from Prussia, Germany. From a young age, Lipmann showed an interest in life sciences and modern art. After receiving a classical education, he studied medicine in Munich and at the University of Königsberg, Berlin, graduating in 1924. He then continued his studies in chemistry at the Kaiser Wilhelm Institute for

Biology in Dahlem, Berlin, where he received a PhD in chemistry in 1928. In 1939, Lipmann emigrated to the US and became a Research Associate in the Department of Biochemistry at Cornell University Medical College in New York. He later joined the Massachusetts General Hospital in Boston as research staff in the Department of Surgery, and then headed his own group in the Biochemical Research Laboratory of that hospital. From 1949 to 1957, he was a professor of biological chemistry at Harvard Medical School, and later taught and conducted research at Rockefeller University in New York City. He became a naturalized citizen in 1944.

Lipmann's primary research interest was in the physiology of organic-bound phosphate and the turnover of metabolic energy in carbohydrate, fatty acid, amino acid, and nucleic acid syntheses and degradations. In 1945, his research culminated in his co-discovery of coenzyme A, for which he shared the Nobel Prize in Physiology and Medicine with German-British physician Hans Adolf Krebs, who was also awarded for his work on the energy-yielding tricarboxylic acid or "Krebs" cycle. Lipmann was also honored with the National Medal of Science in 1966.

Lipmann was recognized with honorary degrees from universities including Copenhagen, Harvard, Paris, Rockefeller, and Yeshiva. He was elected or became an honorary member of many academies of sciences. With his training in medicine and chemistry, Lipmann contributed to laying the foundations of metabolic enzymology as a creative biochemist.

The prostate is a gland in the male reproductive system that has a muscle-driven mechanical function for urination and ejaculation. Located in the pelvis below the bladder, the prostate has the urethra passing through it. It produces a slightly alkaline fluid that is part of semen, a substance emitted during ejaculation and sexual response. The alkaline nature of prostatic fluid helps neutralize the acidity of the vaginal tract, thus prolonging the lifespan of sperm until the time of fertilizing the female egg. Diseases of the prostate include enlargement, inflammation, infection, and cancer, with the latter being the most lethal. Prostate cancer is one of the most common cancers and a significant cause of death among older men. According to the World Health Organization, as of 2012, prostate cancer is the second-most frequently diagnosed cancer and the sixth leading cause of cancer death in males worldwide. In the US, prostate cancer is the third-leading cause of cancer death in men, surpassed by lung and colorectal cancer. More than 80% of men develop prostate cancer by age 80.

One of the most unsettling aspects of prostate cancer is that it often progresses to a serious stage before any symptoms are experienced. When symptoms do occur, they may include urinary frequency, urgency, hesitation, and less commonly, weight loss, retention of urine, or back pain from cancer spread outside of the prostate. High levels of prostate-specific antigen (PSA) are indicative of prostate cancer, making PSA screening crucial for early diagnosis and improving survival rates. Biopsy is the next step in assessing tumor cell activity. Although radiotherapy is sometimes offered as a treatment for prostate cancer, the definitive treatment is prostatectomy, which is nowadays often performed using robotic surgery.

Until the early 1940s, the pharmaceutical influence on advanced prostate cancer was unknown. It wasn't until a Canadian-born surgeon, **Charles Huggins** (1901–1997), showed that chemicals could control the disease. Huggins, born in Halifax, Nova Scotia, to a pharmacist father, attended public schools and received a Bachelor of Arts from Acadia University, Nova Scotia, in 1920. He then moved to the US to study medicine at Harvard Medical School in Boston, where he received his MD in 1924. He completed a surgical residency in general surgery at the University of Michigan and joined the Surgery Department of the University of Michigan, eventually reaching the rank of professor. Huggins conducted cancer research, focusing on the influence of hormone changes on the prostate gland. He discovered that chemical castration by estrogen administration led to gland atrophy, which could be reversed by re-administration of androgen.

In 1941, Huggins and Clarence Hodges recognized the beneficial effect of androgen ablation on metastatic prostate cancer when they treated patients with either castration or estrogen therapy. They monitored prostate size and treatment outcome efficacy by measuring blood prostatic acid phosphatase levels and concluded that androgenic activity in the body influences prostate cancer. Thus, Huggins became the first to use a systemic approach to treat prostate cancer. His research on prostate cancer forever changed physicians' thinking about the behavior of all cancer cells and brought hope for the prospect of treating advanced cancers for the first time. The implications of this discovery reached beyond prostate cancer to other types of cancer, including breast cancer, which he also investigated. Huggins was a leading urologist of his time, and he died in Chicago at the age of 95. A plaque in his office carried his motto: "Discovery is our business."

Huggins won more than 100 awards and honorary degrees from Yale, Acadia, Washington, Leeds, Torino, and Aberdeen Universities, and he was a Fellow of the Royal College of Surgeons and the American College of Surgeons. He also received several other awards from American, British, Scottish, and Italian organizations. In 1966, Huggins shared the Nobel Prize in Physiology or Medicine with virologist Peyton Rous for his research on the relationship between hormones and prostate cancer.

The American phage group was an informal network of biologists that made significant contributions to bacterial genetics and the origins of molecular biology. They took their name from bacteriophages, the bacteria-infecting viruses that devour bacteria and replicate. Using these viruses as a research model, they made discoveries that earned some of them, discussed below, Nobel Laureates.

Understanding the interaction between tumor viruses and the genetic components of cells is important for learning the mechanisms by which viruses cause cancer. This is what **Renato Dulbecco** (1914–2012) did. He was born in Catanzaro, Southern Italy, and spent his childhood in Liguria. After completing his high school education, he moved to the University of Turin and studied mathematics and physics. At the age of 22, he graduated from medical school where he explored morbid anatomy and pathology. There he met two Italians, Salvador Luria, and Rita Levi-Montalcini, who later moved to the US. With their encouragement, Dulbecco would later immigrate to the US. During World War II, Dulbecco was sent to the battlefronts in France and Russia, where he was wounded. After recovering, he joined the resistance against the German occupation. Eventually, he moved, together with Levi-Montalcini, to the US where at Indiana University, he worked with Italian-American **Salvador Luria** on bacteriophages. In 1949, he moved to the California Institute of Technology and joined German-American biophysicist **Max Delbrück** where he became an associate professor and worked on quantitatively assaying animal viruses, including the Western equine encephalitis virus.

In 1962, Dulbecco moved to the Salk Institute, and in 1972, to The Imperial Cancer Research Fund, where he was appointed as a full professor. He then temporarily moved back to Italy where he studied mammary gland cancer stem cells. In 1986, he was among the scientists who launched the Human Genome Project. He returned to the US where he died in La Jolla, California.

Later in his career, Dulbecco was elected to the American Academy of Arts and Sciences and the American Philosophical Society. He was awarded the Marjory Stephenson Prize and Louisa Gross Horwitz Prize from Columbia University. He was also the recipient of the Selman Waksman Award in Microbiology from the National Academy of Sciences. Dulbecco's main achievement was in the late 1950s when he took Howard Temin as a student, and together with David Baltimore, they later shared the 1975 Nobel Prize in Physiology or Medicine for their discoveries of the interaction between tumor viruses and the genetic material of the cell. Specifically, they showed that the transfer of viral genes to the cell is mediated by an enzyme called reverse transcriptase, which replicates the viral genome, in this case made of RNA, into DNA, which is later incorporated into the host genome. Oncoviruses cause some human cancers. Dulbecco's study provided the basis for understanding the molecular mechanisms by which they propagate, thus allowing for better control of them. Dulbecco's discoveries have allowed humans to better understand and fight cancer.

Salvador Luria (1912–1991) was born in Turin, Italy, and attended the medical school at the University of Turin, graduating in 1935. It was there that he met two other future Nobel laureates, Rita Levi-Montalcini, and Renato Dulbecco. For the next two years, Luria served as a medical officer in the Italian army as part of his required service. He then studied radiology at the University of Rome, where he met the German-American biophysicist **Max Delbrück**. Delbrück had established the American Phage Group in the late 1930s, which began to formulate methods for testing genetic theory. In 1945, the Phage Group made substantial progress in unraveling important aspects of genetics that were then mysterious. Other members of the group included Alfred Hershey, Seymour Benzer, James Watson, and Frank Stahl, all of whom were born in the United States, as well as foreign-born scientists such as Salvador Luria, Charles Steinberg, Renato Dulbecco, and **Gunther Stent**, a non-physician biologist born in Germany who worked at the California Institute of Technology in Pasadena, California.

In 1940, Luria fled Mussolini's fascist regime on a bicycle and went to Marseille, where he obtained an immigration visa to the United States with the help of Italian-American physicist **Enrico Fermi**. Luria then received a Rockefeller Foundation fellowship at Columbia University, where he joined Delbrück and Hershey and collaborated on experiments at Vanderbilt University. In his famous Luria-Delbrück experiment in 1943, he demonstrated that inheritance in bacteria must follow Darwinian principles and that mutant bacteria occurring randomly can still bestow viral resistance without the virus being present. This idea of natural selection affecting bacteria has profound consequences, such as explaining how bacteria develop antibiotic resistance.

In 1943, Luria worked at Indiana University, and his first graduate student was James Watson, who later discovered the structure of DNA with Francis Crick. In 1947, Luria became a citizen of the United States. In 1950, he moved to the University of Illinois, where he and Italian microbiologist Giuseppe Bertani discovered the phenomenon of host-controlled restriction, in which bacteria provide a defense against foreign DNA carried by bacteriophages. Later in his career, Luria continued his microbiology and cancer research at MIT in Boston and became an activist and friend of Noam Chomsky and Elie Wiesel, joining them in advocating against nuclear weapon testing and the Vietnam War. Luria died in Lexington, Massachusetts of a heart attack.

Luria won the Nobel Prize in Physiology or Medicine in 1969, along with Max Delbrück and Alfred Hershey, for their discoveries of the replication mechanism and genetic structure of viruses. He also received numerous other awards and recognitions, including the National Medal of Science, membership in the National Academy of Sciences, and serving as president of the American Society for Microbiology. He was awarded the Louisa Gross Horwitz Prize from Columbia University, together with Max Delbrück, and won the 1974 National Book Award in Science for his popular science book "Life: The Unfinished Experiment".

Dendritic cells are a type of antigen-presenting cells that are found in tissues exposed to the external environment, such as the skin, inner lining of the nose, lungs, stomach, and intestines. Recently, they have also been discovered in the blood. Immature dendritic cells can uptake invading pathogens and migrate to the draining lymph nodes. Upon maturation into antigen-presenting cells, they interact with T and B cells to initiate an immune response that defends against invading organisms or tumor cells. Therefore, they are important, as under certain conditions, they may serve as vectors in the immunotherapy of cancer and infectious diseases.

These fascinating dendritic cells were discovered by **Ralph Steinman** (1943-2011), who was born in Montreal, Canada after his family emigrated from Poland. Steinman attended high school in Sherbrooke and received a Bachelor of Science degree from McGill University. After moving to the US, he completed his medical education at Harvard Medical School in 1968 and concluded his internship and residency in internal medicine at Massachusetts General Hospital. In 1970, he joined Rockefeller University in NY, focusing his work particularly on the initiation of immune responses. He soon characterized pathways for the engulfing of molecules by cells, or endocytosis. While working at the laboratory of Zanvil Cohn in 1973 and looking through an electron microscope, he discovered a new type of immune cell with rapidly changing projections, which he called dendritic cells. Steinman recognized that this cell is biochemically distinct from macrophages and could induce T-cell division and initiate killer-T-cell responses to antigens.

Steinman brought scientists from other fields to collaborate with him and was able to make a leap from the bench to the bedside. Through these collaborations, he showed that dendritic cells exist in the blood of humans and, when loaded with antigen, they induce anti-tumor immunity in mice and could be activated by pathogens to initiate immunity.

In 2011, Steinman received one-half of the Nobel Prize in Physiology or Medicine for his discovery of the dendritic cell and its role in adaptive immunity. The other half went to American immunologist Bruce Beutler and German-born French biologist Jules Hoffmann for their discoveries of the activation of innate immunity. The Nobel Prize committee was not aware that Steinman had died three days earlier in Manhattan, NY, from pancreatic cancer. This created a dilemma because the statutes of the Nobel Foundation stipulate that the prize should not be awarded posthumously. However, after deliberation, the committee decided to award him the prize.

Steinman received other awards and recognitions for his lifelong work on dendritic cells, including the Lasker Award for Basic Medical Research, the Gairdner Foundation International Award, and the Cancer Research Institute William Coley Award. He was also made a member of the Institute of Medicine and the National Academy of Sciences. In 2016, the city of Sherbrooke, Quebec, where Steinman lived as a child, named a street rue Ralph Steinman in his honor.

Lasker Award

The Lasker Award is named after **Albert Lasker** (1880–1952), a German immigrant who moved to America with his family in 1840. Lasker grew up in Galveston, Texas and started his career as a newspaper reporter and campaigner for a republican congressman. He later moved to Chicago and worked as an office boy in the Lord and Thomas advertising agency, earning $10 a week. By 1903, his advertising campaigns were successful, and he became a partner in the company. In 1912, he purchased the firm and masterminded a new advertising strategy called "salesmanship in print" that convincingly told consumers why they should buy a product, resulting in astounding success.

In 1904, Lasker and a partner established the 1900 Washer Co. (Whirlpool), which became one of the largest advertising agencies in the nation. In 1908, Lasker played a role in popularizing orange juice in America when Lord & Thomas acquired Sunkist Growers Inc., boosting the citrus consumption and the California orange growers' industry.

Lasker **(Fig 33)** created many successful advertising campaigns, including promoting Lucky Strikes cigarettes for women with the promise that they could stay slender, as well as radio advertising campaigns for Palmolive soap, Pepsodent toothpaste, facial tissue Kleenex, and

Kotex sanitary napkins. He is also credited with creating the soap opera genre and utilizing radio and television as media driven by advertising. Lasker revolutionized the advertising industry, fundamentally changed popular culture, and became known as the "father of modern advertising."

In 1916, Lasker owned the Chicago Cubs baseball team and, along with German American sports executive Charles Weeghman, moved the Cubs to their current home—which became known as Wrigley Field. In 1925, Lasker sold the team to his minor partner, William Wrigley Jr. After the Great Depression, Lasker donated one of his private estates, Mill Road Farm in Lake Forest, Illinois, which included a golf course, to the University of Chicago.

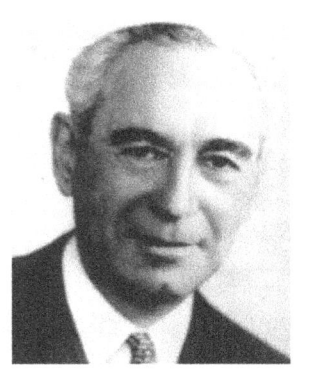

Fig 33. Immigrant philanthropist Albert Lasker was "father of modern advertising" with his wife Mary supported the American Cancer Society and established the Lasker Foundation, offering the Lasker Awards. (Texas State Historical Association)

Lasker used his persuasive advertising skills to help the Republican Party by utilizing modern advertising techniques to sell their candidates. He was a key advisor in the 1920 Warren Harding campaign, which targeted advertising towards women who had recently gained the right to vote. In return, President Harding appointed Lasker as chairman of the US Shipping Board.

In 1940, Lasker married his third wife Mary Woodard, a wealthy owner of a mass-produced clothing business who had previous encounters with illness. When Mary's mother had a stroke and there was no treatment available, Mary was incensed by the lack of medical knowledge to cure her mother, who eventually died from the disease. Mary's mission became eradicating disease, and the couple became nationally prominent philanthropists who sponsored medicine and used their extensive network and social connections to play key roles in promoting and expanding the National Institutes of Health.

In 1943, the Laskers waged war against disease and cancer. They donated to the financially struggling American Society for Cancer Control and used an advertising campaign to raise funds for the organization. Albert later joined its board, and in 1945, the society flourished and was renamed the American Cancer Society. With Mary's persistence, they raised funds for medical research and founded the Lasker Foundation, which offers the Lasker Awards. With her husband's support, Mary became known as "the fairy godmother of medical research". Ironically, Albert developed colon cancer, and despite surgery, his disease could not be eradicated. He was confined to a hospital bed, waiting for death from a disease he had tried to conquer, and he died in New York at the age of 72. Lasker was voted into the American National Business Hall of Fame.

The Lasker Award was established in 1942 and has been awarded annually since 1945 to living persons who have made substantial contributions to medical science or who have performed public service on behalf of medicine. The Awards are administered by the Albert and Mary Lasker Foundation, headquartered in New York City. The award is often referred to as "America's Nobel" and recognizes the contributions of scientists, physicians, and public servants who have made major advances towards knowledge, diagnosis, treatment, cure, and prevention of human disease. In doing so, Albert and Mary Lasker established a legacy of advocacy and philanthropy in support of science and health. The Lasker Award has gained a reputation for identifying future winners of the Nobel Prize, with eighty-six Lasker laureates receiving the Nobel Prize, including thirty-two in the last two decades.

There are four categories for Lasker Awards: Basic Research, Clinical Research, Special Achievement, and Public Service. The Basic and Clinical Awards are given annually, while the Special Achievement and Public Service Awards are given in alternate years. The Basic Medical Research Award is dedicated to discoveries that open new areas of biomedical science, while the Clinical Medical Research Award is offered for advances that improve the lives and health of people. The Special Achievement Award in Medical Science is given for research accomplishments that engender a feeling of awe and respect, and the Public Service Award is bestowed for improving the public's understanding of medical research, public health, or healthcare, serving as a spokesperson for medical research or public health, and providing outstanding public health practice.

Since inaugurating the first award in 1946 until 2019, approximately 395 individuals have been awarded the Lasker Awards, and as of 2018, around 61 immigrants have won the Award. Several non-physician immigrant scientists have won the Lasker Award over the years for their contributions in the medical field. A brief discussion of these contributions is apropos.

The Canadian-American journalist **Catherine MacKenzie** (1894–1949) was awarded a Lasker in 1947 for her work on mental illness. **Choh Hao Li** (1913–1987), a Chinese-American biochemist, went on to receive the 1962 Lasker for successfully isolating and synthesizing the human pituitary growth hormone. **Günter Blobel** (1936–2018), a German-American biologist, won the 1993 Lasker and the 1999 Nobel for showing how cell proteins have a "virtual ZIP code" that directs them to where they should be. **Miguel Ondetti** (1930-2004), an Argentinian-American chemist, was honored with the Lasker in 1999 for developing Captopril, a drug that helped patients around the globe with high blood pressure and chronic heart failure.

Between 2000 and 2019, ten other immigrants were recipients of the Lasker. **Alexander Varshavsky**, a Russian-American biochemist, won the 2000 award for his discovery of ubiquitination, a system that regulates protein degradation—which influences cell cycle, malignant transformation, and responses to inflammation and immunity. **Oliver Smithies** (1925–2017), a British-American biochemist, and **Mario Capecchi**, an Italian-American geneticist, both received the 2001 Lasker for manipulating the mouse genome and creating a genetically-modified "knock-out mouse," which today serves as a model for many human diseases. Capecchi was also a co-winner of the 2007 Nobel Prize in Physiology or Medicine.

Jack Szostak, a Canadian-American biologist, and **Elizabeth Blackburn**, an Australian-American, won 2006 Lasker awards for their discovery of telomerase, an RNA-containing enzyme that synthesizes the ends of chromosomes, protecting them and the integrity of the genome. Both were also 2009 Nobel Prize laureates for the same work. **Napoleone Ferrara**, an Italian-American molecular biologist, won 2010 award for discovering VEGF, a mediator of angiogenesis and the development of an effective anti-VEGF therapy for macular degeneration, a leading cause of blindness in the elderly.

Thomas Südhof, a German-American biochemist, won the 2013 award for discoveries of molecular machinery and regulatory mechanisms that influence rapid release of neurotransmitters. **Peter Walter**, a German-American molecular biologist, won the 2014 award for discovery of unfolded protein systems that detect harmful proteins in the endoplasmic reticulum and signal for the nucleus to carry out corrective measures. **Michael Hall** is a Swiss-American who won the 2017 award for discovery of certain nutrient-activated proteins and their central role in the metabolic control of cell growth. Lastly, **Michael Grunstein**, a Romanian-born immigrant, won the 2018 Lasker for showing how gene expression is influenced by chemical modification of proteins that package DNA within chromosomes.

Three notable immigrant physicians who were discussed in detail previously, won the Lasker awards. **Georgios Papanikolaou** (1883–1962) was a Greek-American physician who won in 1950 for his pioneering work in cytopathology and invention of the "pap smear" which detects early cervical cancer.

A historical Lasker Award was won by **Paul Brand**, the British immigrant Orthopedic Surgeon, who won the Lasker in 1960 for his work in rehabilitation of the disabled and treating leprosy patients in India and the US.

Philip Levine (1900–1987) a Russian-American physician who was eight years old when his family escaped Tsarist Russia to America and settled in Brooklyn, New York. In 1923, Levine received a medical degree from Cornell University Medical School. In 1925, he became assistant to Austrian-American **Karl Landsteiner** at the Rockefeller Institute and later took up research work with the bacteriophage program at the University of Wisconsin-Madison. The importance of Levine's work was recognized with a Lasker in 1946 as he was the first to suggest that Rh antibodies made by a pregnant mother which can be the cause of a fatal newborn anemia.

Two living immigrant physicians were recent recipients of a Lasker. **Eric Kandel**, an Austrian-American physician and neuroscientist, was the recipient of the 1983 Lasker and shared the Nobel Prize in 2000 with two others for his research on memory and the physiological basis of memory storage in neurons. **Rachel Schneerson**, a Polish-born physician, she is best known for her development of the vaccine for Haemophiles Influenza B, for which she received Lasker in 1996.

In her op-ed of 2018, Lasker's President, Claire Pomeroy stated that immigrant Laureates "open doors and create opportunity for sometimes unforeseen medical science brilliance to flourish, and when that happens, we all benefit."

Pulitzer Prize

The man behind the famed prize is **Joseph Pulitzer** (1847–1911), whose story is captivating. Pulitzer was a Hungarian-born American journalist, politician, and philanthropist. He grew up in Budapest, Hungary, to a height of 6 feet one inch, speaking German and French and devouring books. When his wealthy Jewish father died, the family became impoverished. Pulitzer struggled to enlist in different European armies for sustenance but to no avail. In response to an advertisement by the US government for volunteers to serve in the Union Army during the Civil War in 1864, Pulitzer, at the age of 17, lied about his age being 20 and boarded a ship of male recruits. After six weeks at sea, he reached Boston Harbor.

During the war not many young men volunteered to serve especially the children of wealthy people. Pulitzer was able to join the army and earned $200 at enrollment. He served in the 1st Lincoln Cavalry established by German-American revolutionary **Carl Schurz**. After the war ended and having served in the army for eight months, Pulitzer returned to New York homeless, sleeping in the cobbled streets. He hitched in a boxcar to Mark Twain's city of St Louis and worked in a stable and lumberyard. Later, he worked in a restaurant that was frequented by members of the St Louis philosophical Society, including the Scottish-American philosopher and lecturer **Thomas Davidson** (1840–1900). Pulitzer was thought to have had an intimate relationship with Thomas Davidson during this period.

Pulitzer **(Fig 34)** spoke German, French and Hungarian—but little English. He became a member of the society and began visiting a local library where he read extensively with a special interest in philosophy books. His English improved and he began writing articles for small newspapers. One of his earlier publications was a story about someone who cheated him out of five dollars.

Pulitzer later studied law and became a reporter for the German language newspaper *Westliche Post*, partly owned by Carl Schurz. He now associated with intellectuals, including **Joseph Keppler** (1838–1894), an Austrian-born American cartoonist and caricaturist, who influenced the growth of satirical cartooning in the US.

In 1878, Pulitzer established the *St Louis Post Dispatch*. He became wealthy and influential and helped Schurz to be elected as senator. He moved to New York and established *The New York World* newspaper, which was published from 1860 until 1931 and played a major role in American history as a leading voice of the Democratic Party. Initially, Pulitzer adopted yellow journalism for his newspaper to survive the competitive environment especially with William Hurst. Later, Pulitzer changed course and hired some quality reporters.

Pulitzer was elected as a congressman for New York and became a leading figure in the Democratic Party. Later, he returned to his journalistic work. One of the reporters who was working for Pulitzer was Nellie Bly. As an undercover reporter, she pretended to have a mental disorder and exposed the terrible treatment the mentally ill received at the Woman's Lunatic Asylum. In doing so, Pulitzer and Bly established the new field of investigative journalism. Pulitzer's newspaper became the largest newspaper in the country. It was a powerful instrument for reform that elected presidents, helped politicians win elections, sent corrupt statesmen to jail, and articulated public aspirations and demands.

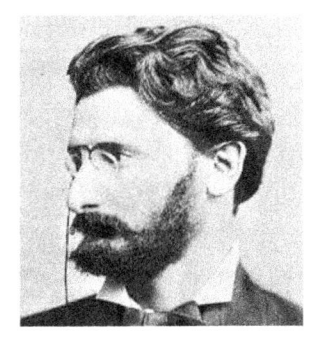

Fig 34. Hungarian-born American journalist, politician, and philanthropist Joseph Pulitzer was founder of Columbia School of Journalism and Pulitzer Foundation. (The Pulitzer Prizes)

In January 1884, the construction of the Statue of Liberty was completed in Paris but remained there for one year waiting for its pedestal to be finished in New York City. Wealthy New Yorkers did not want to donate the $100,000 necessary to complete this pedestal. Joseph Pulitzer wrote in his national newspaper *The World* an article admonishing the many "stingy millionaires" in New York who would not donate the money to complete the pedestal. In a series of articles, he offered his own contribution and encouraged others to give small donations—in return, he would list their names in the newspaper. With the help of Pulitzer's ingenious initiative, everyday Americans raised the money needed, and the pedestal was completed in 1886.

In 1892, Pulitzer founded the Columbia School of Journalism with a major donation, which opened in 1912. The Pulitzer Prize was then established posthumously in 1917, through provisions in his will. The prize is an annual award administered by Columbia University in New York City and has been given to recipients since 1918 and continues to be given annually to recognize and reward excellence in American journalism, photography, literature, history, poetry, music, and drama. Today, Pulitzer is more known for the prize that bears his name than his other important contributions to the literary world. Just as the Scottish-American **Andrew Carnegie** gave America mass knowledge through libraries, Pulitzer gave America the mass media.

Pulitzer Prizes are usually awarded to an American author or organization and offered in twenty-one different categories. The winner receives a certificate and a $15,000 cash award; the winning news organization in the public service category receives a gold medal. The authors may be candidates who submit their work for the competition or nominees selected by a nominating group for their contribution. The Pulitzer Prize Board selects one winner from the three finalists in each category.

The Pulitzer Prize does not have a category for medical achievements, but prizes have been awarded over the years to physicians and topics related to healthcare. This includes subjects like medical malpractice issues, epidemics, and new treatments. An example of such reporting on an epidemic is Laurie Garrett, who won the Pulitzer in 1996 for reporting from Zaire on the Ebola virus outbreak.

Books focusing on medical issues have been awarded the prize and one of the earliest physicians to earn the prize was Harvey Cushing, the neurosurgeon and pathologist. Cushing received his medical degree from Harvard Medical School and practiced at Johns Hopkins Hospital in Baltimore, winning a Pulitzer in 1926 for his book *The Life of Sir William Osler*. This biography portrays Osler as a brilliant, innovative teacher and physician who revolutionized the art of practicing medicine at a patient's bedside. The book vividly illustrates the times

Osler inhabited, the evolution of modern medicine, the training of doctors, holistic medical thought, and the doctor-patient relationship.

Several other books have won a Pulitzer and were written by immigrant Americans. The sociologist Paul Starr won a Pulitzer in 1984 for his book *The Social Transformation of American Medicine* (1982), which is about medicine and healthcare in the US. It examines the evolution and culture of medicine from the colonial period through the last quarter of the twentieth century. It details the attempts of the AMA to improve academic training of physicians, the general standard of professional medical practice, and the professional status of physicians. Medical historian David M Oshinsky won a Pulitzer in 2006 for his book *Polio: An American Story* (2005) that documented the polio epidemic in the US during the 1940s and 1950s and the race to develop a vaccine. In 2011, Indian-American physician Siddhartha Mukherjee was also awarded a Pulitzer for *The Emperor of All Maladies: A Biography of Cancer* (2010), a detailed history of cancer.

The Pulitzer Awards continued to be bestowed on immigrants. Since 1917, an estimated 61 immigrants have won the Pulitzer Prize and the first immigrant to receive a prize was in 1976, fifty-nine years after the foundation was established upon the bequest of immigrant Joseph Pulitzer.

The Carnegie Corporation of New York, established by immigrant **Andrew Carnegie** in 1911, to promote knowledge, recognized thirty-four "Great Immigrants" in 2022, from thirty-two countries. They enriched and strengthened our nation through their contributions and actions in many fields. Some of those are physicians, and others are women.

The next chapter will explore the contributions of women physicians to the medical field with emphasis on those who ventured from their foreign birthplace to our shores and enhanced American medicine.

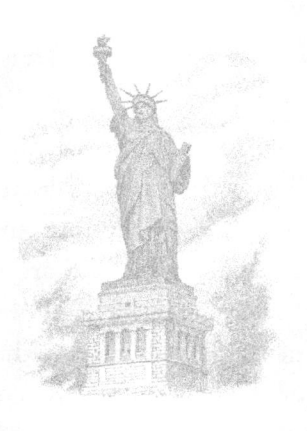

CHAPTER 10

Women Physicians

Long before medicine became a profession, primary care-givers were often female. Women provided medical care for centuries as apothecaries, herbalists, village healers, wise women, and especially as midwives. During the reign of Henry V (1413–1422), it was outlawed for women to practice medicine in England. Between 1400 and 1700, the medieval church in Europe branded wise women as witches, and more than 100,000 women healers (including nuns) were put to trial and 60,000 burned at the stake.

Women nevertheless maintained a monopoly on delivering babies until the early 17th century, when midwifery began to change from a female to a male occupation. The transition was not smooth and began in 1522, when Dr Wertt of Hamburg dressed up as a woman to observe midwives during childbirth. However, when his gender was discovered, he was burned alive while other physicians watched. Louis XIV, King of France, used male midwives to deliver the illegitimate children of his mistresses. The practice of male midwives subsequently began to gain acceptance later in the mid-sixteenth century, and the foundation was laid for men's work as obstetricians. British surgeon Peter Chamberlen (1560-1631) invented the obstetrical forceps that aid in delivering the newborn's head, a device that midwives previously did not use. In the past, the objection toward male midwifes came from husbands who believed it inappropriate for their wives to be exposed to men, while women often thought a male midwife could never understand the pains of labor. One ritual among Mexican Indigenous communities was to tie a string around the husband's testicles so the wife could pull the string with every contraction and ensures the man felt her pain. Even today, many women prefer to have female obstetricians delivering their children.

James Barry (1789-1865) was a surgeon in the British Army, who obtained a medical degree from the University of Edinburgh, then served in many parts of the British Empire and rose to the rank of Inspector General in charge of military hospitals, the second-highest medical office in the British Army. Barry improved conditions for many wounded soldiers and those of native inhabitants and performed the first recorded caesarean section by a European in Africa. Upon his death a maid was laying out his body, discovered that he was a woman whose gender was confirmed by a post-mortem examination. Later it was determined that Doctor Barry was born Margaret Ann Bulkley and known as female during childhood but chosen to live her adult life as a man to be accepted as medical student and pursue a career as a surgeon in a male dominated profession.

Women continued to face obstacles to becoming physicians until the 19th century when gradual change began to occur. Women's struggle and the suffrage movement in America ensued in 1848, at the Seneca Falls Convention in New York which paved the way, among other things, for women to receive educational opportunities, including enrollment in medical schools.

Immigrant Physician Suffragettes

Foreign-born physician women joined the suffrage movement advocating for women's economic, educational, and voting rights. We know only of a few of them, however.

Anna Shaw (1847–1919) came to the US at the age of four and settled with her family in Michigan. She enrolled in the School of Theology at Boston University and became a Methodist minister. She then pursued a medical education at Boston University and received a medical degree in 1886. She was not content with ministering and healing, and thus became a speaker for temperance and women's suffrage, traveling the length and breadth of the country to give hundreds of lectures. Despite her being an immigrant, however, she did not support immigrant women and was a nativist.

A Chinese-born American female physician also joined the suffrage movement in the US, but unlike Shaw she actively supported immigrant women's rights. **Me-Iung Ting** (1891-1969) was 15 when her father arranged her marriage, of which she did not approve. With her brother's help she escaped China to the US, attended college, and later graduated from University of Michigan Medical School, Ann Arbor in 1920, the only Chinese woman in her class. She returned to China, married, and practiced medicine, becoming the director of Peiyang Women's Hospital in Tientsin. She occasionally revisited the US but later emigrated permanently in 1950 to escape the communist regime. For the remainder of her career, Ting **(Fig 35)** continued her contribution to medicine in Florida and Mississippi through charity work, but also labored relentlessly to improve medical care for women, children, and refugees, even when it put her at great personal risk. Ting's experience, first as a foreign student studying in the US, and later as an immigrant- American physician helping women with their health and humanity, illustrate the possibilities of American medical education and legal immigration.

Another Chinese-born woman with no less influence than Ting on the suffrage movement was **Mabel Lee** (1896–1966) who emigrated with her mother in 1900 to reunite with her father who had emigrated earlier and worked as a minister in Washington State—men often emigrated before the family. Her family then settled in New York City China Town in 1905. Like her father, Lee became a minister but later studied economics. She began her involvement in the suffrage movement at a very early age, writing essays and leading parades in New York City, including the Chinese-American women's parade. While in college, Lee began writing articles calling for gender equality and giving speeches. Lee was able to mobilize the Chinese community in America to support women's right to vote. Though women did win the right to vote in the state of New York in 1917, Lee still could not exercise her right to vote because of The Chinese Exclusion Act, which did not consider Chinese immigrants as citizens.

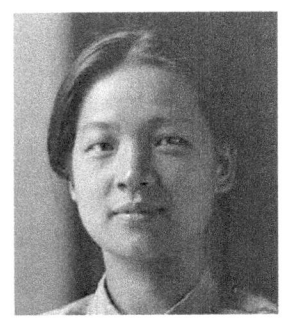

Fig 35. Chinese immigrant physician Me-Iung Ting joined the suffrage movement, besides her charity work, she labored relentlessly to improve medical care for women, children, and refugees. (Wikipedia)

American Influence on British Women's Medical Education

In Great Britain, women like Elizabeth Garrett Anderson and Sophia Jex-Blake were inspired by American women who began graduating from medical schools and struggling for acceptance as physicians in the medical profession. They encountered opposition from other professors in medical schools, from medical students, and from the public. Educators expressed concerns that, as women, they were incapable of handling the rigorous demand of the medical curriculum. Medical students objected to a mingling of the sexes in medical schools, which were male-only dominions. Public opinion was also against women joining the British medical field due to the belief that a woman's place was at home, besides their lacking the intellect and judgment of men. Some even suggested that workingwomen would lead to an increase in celibacy among men who become deprived of sex while women were working away from home.

In 1858, in a coastal English town, a 21-year-old American-born Elizabeth Garrett Anderson (1836-1917) was reading an article in the *English Woman's Journal* about Elizabeth Blackwell, the first woman doctor who had graduated nine years earlier in the US. A year later, Blackwell visited London and gave lectures encouraging women to become doctors. Garret attended Blackwell's lectures and met her afterward, later corresponding with her by letter. Blackwell was a great influence on Garrett, who decided to follow Blackwell's example and attain a British medical degree. She also faced obstacles as Blackwell had in America and had to first work as a nurse. She applied to Oxford, Cambridge, Glasgow, and Edinburgh universities before finally being accepted in Edinburgh. Elizabeth Garrett Anderson was the first woman to qualify in Britain as a physician.

Sophia Jex-Blake (1840-1912) was an English physician and feminist who led a campaign to secure women's access to medical education in Edinburgh, later becoming the first practicing female doctor in Scotland. In 1865, before commencing her medical education and shortly after the end of the American Civil War, Sophia had visited Boston to learn about women's education and assisted Lucy Sewell who had graduated from New England Female Medical College at a time when other women were already claiming medical degrees. Sophia worked at the New England Hospital for Women and Children. She was strongly influenced by the co-educational approach in the US and later published *A Visit to Some American Schools and Colleges*. She returned to England and was admitted to Edinburgh University as part of a group of seven women students despite the opposition of Joseph

Lister and other physicians. These seven Edinburgh students faced prejudice inside and outside the classroom, and even when they completed all their courses, they were denied graduation by the university. In 1874, the London school of medicine for women opened with an inaugural class of 14 students, including Sophia, who after graduation moved to Scotland and became Scotland's first practicing woman doctor. As we will see later, a British-born American woman helped establish the first London School of Medicine for Women in England.

Immigrant Women Physicians

In the early 19th century United States, the prejudice against women seeking formal medical education forced many instead to seek alternative practices such as herbs and hydrotherapy. However, American women led the way in winning the right to attend medical schools. Consequently, the first-year class of medical students at Johns Hopkins medical school had fifteen men and three women. The second year, 40 students were admitted, eight of who were women.

So, who were those pioneer women who wrestled against their gender prejudice to become physicians? Were there any immigrants among them? No doubt there were many, but we know of only a handful and will chronicle those who made history trying, beginning with one who shattered the taboo against women's right to a medical education.

Elizabeth Blackwell (1821-1910) was born British but blossomed as an American. She emigrated in 1832 with her family from Britain and grew up in Cincinnati as one of nine children. She settled in Philadelphia at a time when medicine was still a dreadful business involving terrible practices. Calomel was considered a miracle cure and used in mega doses as a panacea for all ailments. Later, it was realized that the mercury it contained had a poisonous effect, and its use was abandoned. Blackwell's interest in medicine and desire to change prevailing practices compelled her to study anatomy privately. Blackwell worked as a teacher and governess. While in South Carolina teaching music, she had access to the medical library of Dr Samuel Dickson and engrossed herself in his medical books, which solidified her interest in medicine. She was influenced by the book *Woman in the Nineteenth Century* (1845) by Margaret Fuller.

Some women at the time did train as apprentices to experienced doctors to become unlicensed physicians. Blackwell was discouraged by friends and neighbors due to the strong opposition at the time. Blackwell nevertheless attempted to enter several American medical schools but was repeatedly rejected. The reason given, as in Britain, was that women were intellectually inferior and ill-suited to medicine. She was advised to disguise herself as a man, but she refused. She was told to instead seek a medical education in Europe, but things were no better there. Finally, in 1847, the same year the AMA was established, she was accepted at Geneva Medical College, today, Hobart College, in New York.

As a medical student, Blackwell faced obstacles in being barred from certain classes and harassed by male students. Professors forced her to sit apart at lectures and excluded her from attending laboratories. Even townspeople shunned her as a "bad" woman for defying her gender role. Nevertheless, the historical breakthrough came when against all odds in 1849, Blackwell became the first woman to graduate from a medical school in the US; not only that, but she graduated at the top of her class.

During the American Civil War, Blackwell **(Fig 36)** and her sister aided in medical efforts and trained nurses in hospitals. She was a sympathizer with the North and the anti-slavery movement. She became a friend of Florence Nightingale and preceptor to Marie Zakrzewska helping her pursue

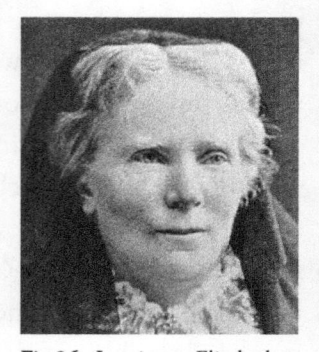

Fig 36. Immigrant Elizabeth Blackwell was the first woman to graduate from an American medical school in 1847, establish the first medical college for women in New York City and helped establish the first London School of Medicine for Women in England. (Library of Congress)

a medical education. In 1857, with the help of Zakrzewska and Quaker friends, Blackwell established the 'New Infirmary for Indigent Women and Children' in New York City. In 1868, Blackwell established her own medical college for women in New York City, thus opening the doors of opportunity for those excluded from medical training in a male dominated profession. Finally, she went to England and along with others including Nightingale and Thomas Huxley, Blackwell helped establish the first London School of Medicine for Women in England. In 1895, Blackwell published her autobiography *Pioneer Work in Opening the Medical Profession to Women*. National Women Physicians' Day in the US is on February 3rd in celebration of Blackwell's birthday.

Another immigrant who collaborated with Blackwell in fighting prejudice against women physicians and changed the face of medicine itself is **Marie Zakrzewska** (1829-1902), who was born in Germany to a midwife mother and a noble but impoverished Polish father who had lost all his wealth to Russia. Her father did not allow her to pursue study so she left school at the age of 13. Her mother's career sparked her interest in medicine, and she read any medicinal book that she could find. First, she attended a midwifery school in Berlin and then followed in her mother's footsteps; she excelled and became a professor at the same college. She then studied medicine and decided to emigrate to America for better opportunities, not knowing the challenges American women physicians were still experiencing.

In 1853, Zakrzewska **(Fig 37)** and her sister landed in New York where she yearned to have the opportunity to become a physician, only to realize that female physicians faced considerable disadvantages in the US. Impoverished, she took a temporary job as a seamstress earning a dollar a day. One year

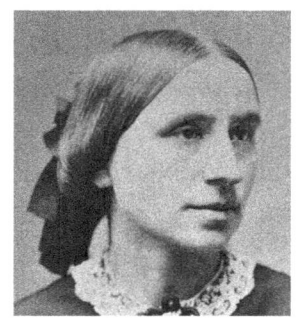

Fig 37. Immigrant Marie Zakrzewska, opened in Boston the New England Hospital for Women and Children, which was the first to provide gynecological and obstetrical care and formal nursing education. (Public domain)

later, she was introduced to Elizabeth Blackwell and joined her dispensary. In order to obtain a license to practice medicine in the US, she attended the Western Reserve University medical program with Blackwell's encouragement, where she was one of four women among two hundred male students. Despite hostility and appeals for her dismissal, she persevered and successfully graduated in 1856.

Upon graduation, it was not easy for her to practice in New York, even with a medical degree. She faced the same hostility from a male controlled profession and was ostracized by the public; therefore, she and Blackwell first opened an office in Blackwell's house to practice medicine. By 1857, they had established the New York Infirmary for Women and Children, which became a success. Zakrzewska, moved to Boston, a city with less prejudice against women physicians than New York City. She became a professor of Obstetrics and Diseases of Women and Children at Boston Female Medical College. In 1862, she opened the New England Hospital for Women and Children, which was the first in Boston to provide gynecological and obstetrical care; it was also the first in America to offer formal education in nursing. Most importantly, it offered an opportunity for women physicians to practice. The facility expanded and Mary Jacobi also joined the hospital, which treated the poor for free and relied entirely on donations.

Despite her success, Zakrzewska was denied admission to medical organizations. After repeated efforts along with her women colleagues, she finally succeeded in convincing Johns Hopkins University to open its doors to women for medical training. After retirement, she became a feminist and abolitionist. The first black nurse in America graduated from Zakrzewska's school in 1879. Zakrzewska also introduced the German idea of building sand gardens for children to America, beginning in the city of Boston. Zakrzewska died in Jamaica Plain in Massachusetts. Her home lies on the Boston Women Heritage Trail.

Besides the struggles Blackwell and Zakrzewska endured to become physicians, they also helped others to overcome those same obstacles and receive medical training. One such person was **Mary Jacobi** (1842–1906) who was born in London and moved with her parents to America in 1848. She grew up in New York, where after finishing school, she studied Greek, science, and medicine privately with Elizabeth Blackwell and others. In 1863, she became the first woman to graduate from a US school of pharmacy.

Jacobi **(Fig 21)** graduated from the Women's Medical College of Pennsylvania and joined Zakrzewska in practicing medicine, founding the New England Hospital for Women and Children in Boston in 1862. She served in the Civil War as a medical aid. She then further advanced her medical education by studying in Paris, France. Back in the US, she conducted research and became a professor at the new Women's Medical College of the New York Infirmary and Mount Sinai Hospital. She then organized the Association for the Advancement of the Medical Education of Women in 1872. She married **Abraham Jacobi**, a German-American physician who is now known as the "father of American pediatrics." She won the Boylston Prize from Harvard University for an influential paper where she refuted the supposed physical limitations of women during menstruation, which made them allegedly ill-suited for education.

In 1886, Jacobi opened a children's ward at the New York Infirmary. In 1894, she wrote *Common Sense Applied to Women's Suffrage*, which was later reprinted and used to build the women's suffrage movement in the US. She was a prolific medical writer, publishing 9 books and over 120 scientific papers; and before her death, Jacobi wrote a detailed report of her own fatal brain tumor, "Description of the Early Symptoms of the Meningeal Tumor Compressing the Cerebellum." Prominent physicians, including William Osler and Emily Blackwell, attended her funeral in New York. In 1993, Jacobi was inducted into the National Women's Hall of Fame.

Anna Shaw (1847-1919) was an immigrant activist and Methodist minister. Shaw was born in Newcastle, England, and as a child she emigrated with her family to the US, first settling in Lawrence, Massachusetts, and later on the frontiers of Michigan. Her father was engaged in the Abolitionist movement; he and her brother joined the Civil War effort, while she supported the family, working first as a teacher and later a seamstress, all while studying in high school.

Shaw became a preacher and entered college in a Methodist school, which led her later to become one of the first ordained female Methodist ministers in the US. Following ordination, she graduated from Boston University Medical School in 1886. During her medical school years, she became an outspoken advocate of women's rights, involved in the American Woman Suffrage Association. After meeting Susan B Anthony, Shaw joined the National Woman Suffrage Association and was instrumental in merging the two associations creating a united suffrage movement, the National American Woman Suffrage Association—and became the president of that association for eleven years. When the association adopted more militant tactics, Shaw resigned her position as the president.

During World War I, Shaw was head of the Women's Committee of the US Council of National Defense. For her service, she was the first woman to earn the Distinguished Service Medal. She continued to campaign for women's suffrage until her death in Moylan, Pennsylvania. She gave over 10,000 speeches, but her 1915 speech "The Fundamental Principle of a Republic" became one of American Rhetoric's Top Speeches of the 20th Century. Shaw was recognized posthumously in 2000 and inducted into the National Women's Hall of Fame. In 2020, she was named an honoree of the National Women's History Alliance. Two women's centers, one in Albion College and another in Boston University School of Theology, as well as a high school in Philadelphia were all named after her. A statue was erected in her image in Big Rapids, Michigan.

By the beginning of the 20th century, women in the US no longer experienced the same hurdles in getting into medical schools. Women physicians focused their energy instead on providing exceptionally innovative and specialized medical care. The following five immigrant women exemplify the creativity displayed by this new generation as a result.

The first woman to become Nobel laureate was the Polish Marie Curie who won a prize for physics in 1903. As of 2021, 59 Nobel Prizes have been awarded to 58 women internationally. Twenty of those women were Americans. Twelve women won prizes in the category of Physiology and Medicine, and eight of those were Americans. However, the first American woman to win a prize for Physiology and Medicine was an immigrant called **Gerty Cori** (1896–1957) who was born in Prague. Cori was born into a Jewish family but converted to Catholicism and grew up in Vienna. At the age of 16, she decided to be a physician. With the encouragement of her uncle, a professor of pediatrics, she attended a medical school in Prague, and in 1920, she graduated alongside her husband **Carl Cori** (1896–1984).

In Vienna, Gerty focused her career on pediatrics and blood diseases. Because of increasing anti-Semitism, she emigrated in 1922 to the US, becoming a naturalized citizen in 1928. Gerty began her career in the US with medical research for the study of malignant diseases in Buffalo, New York and collaborated with Carl on most of her research, especially on carbohydrate metabolism. Later, they moved to Washington University in St Louis Missouri, where both conducted further biochemistry research focusing on glycogen. She and her husband discovered the glucose 1-phosphate compound that breaks down glycogen, which is now known as the Cori ester, and they identified the enzyme phosphorylase that catalyzed its chemical formation. Gerty also studied glycogen storage disease.

For their discovery of the process of catalytic conversion of glycogen, a process known as the Cori cycle, she and her husband won the Nobel Prize in 1947. Gerty received numerous awards and acknowledgments. President Harry Truman appointed her as board member to the National Science Foundation. The US Postal Service released a stamp with her image in 2008. Gerty developed myelosclerosis, a bone marrow disease most probably caused by exposure to X-ray radiation during her research and she died ten years later.

Caused by uterine contractions and pressure on the cervix, labor pain of vaginal delivery, during childbirth, is one of the most severe pains to be experienced. About 60% of women giving birth at hospitals receive epidural anesthesia for pain relief. The procedure is done by injecting anesthetic with a long needle placed in the lower back within the epidural space that contains spinal fluid around the spinal cord. A German born anesthesiologist, in the 1950s, developed a special needle used for epidural anesthesia and was instrumental in introducing and popularizing the use of epidural anesthesia during delivery. **Gertie Marx** (1912–2004) was born in Frankfurt, and attended medical school at the University of Frankfurt, but completed her medical education in 1937, at the University of Bern, Switzerland. In 1937, she escaped, Nazi Germany, and emigrated to the US, settling in NY New York City.

In 1940, Marx became the first resident in the anesthesiology residency program at Beth Israel Hospital. In 1943, she joined the anesthesia attending staff at that same hospital. She then moved to Albert Einstein College of Medicine where she would remain until retirement in 1995. Marx focused her six-decade-long career on obstetric anesthesiology, and the anesthetic needs of pregnant women, despite facing early opposition as a medical professional for being a woman. In the 1950s, she pioneered the use of epidural analgesia during childbirth, which benefited women worldwide. She also recognized that hypotension is a common complication of the technique and recommended giving intravenous fluid as a prophylactic measure. Max became known as "the mother of obstetric anesthesia." She developed the Gertie Marx Spinal Needle, which is less damaging to the spinal cord. Marx is credited with developing obstetric anesthesia as a specialty and was also a founding editor of the quarterly *Obstetric Anesthesia Digest*.

She received several awards, and Queen Elizabeth II of England later presented her with a lifetime service medal from the Royal College of Anaesthetists in 1993.

A catastrophic medical blunder hit Europe in the 1950s when the Thalidomide drug was introduced to the market by a German pharmaceutical company. It was prescribed for women's morning sickness during early pregnancy. Thousands of women took the drug, which was marketed in more than 40 countries, but in November 1961, the drug was withdrawn after the discovery that it was causing severe fetal deformities. Thalidomide is estimated to have caused the death of about 2,000 children and serious birth defects in more than 10,000 children—with over half of them in West Germany. The thalidomide tragedy has become the greatest prescription disaster in medical history.

The FDA did not authorize Thalidomide for marketing and distribution in the US. Thanks to the courage and perseverance of one Canadian-American physician who resisted repeated pressure from big Pharma to approve the drug, thus saving countless children from potential catastrophe. That was **Francis Kelsey** (1914–2015) who received her degree in Pharmacology in Canada, later accepting a position at the Pharmacology Department at the University of Chicago. While studying for her PhD in Pharmacology, she assisted in research sponsored by the FDA, which uncovered 107 deaths caused by the solvent diethylene glycol. Kelsey developed an interest in teratogens, drugs that cause congenital birth defects. In 1950, she received a medical degree from the University of Chicago, began to practice medicine and taught pharmacology in South Dakota. While in Chicago working on a synthetic cure for malaria, she also learned that some drugs could pass through the placental barrier reaching the developing embryo of an unborn child.

In the 1950s, Kelsey **(Fig 38)** became a US citizen and by 1960 was hired by the FDA in Washington DC. One of her first assignments was to review an application from Richardson Merrell for the drug thalidomide to be prescribed to pregnant women for morning sickness across the US. Although the drug was already approved in Canada, along with 20 European and African countries, Kelsey withheld approval of the drug and requested further studies. Her concern was that the inadequately tested drug could pass the placenta affecting the embryo. Despite continuing pressure from Thalidomide's manufacturer, Kelsey persisted in requesting additional safety information to prove the drug was not harmful to the fetus.

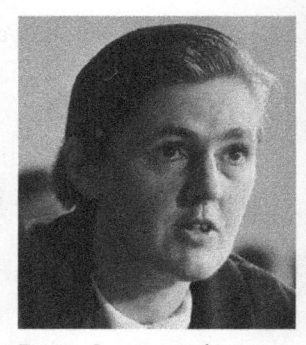

Fig 38. Immigrant physician Francis Kelsey averted US tragedy similar to that in Europe that caused newborn birth defects, by not approving the use of Thalidomide drug for pregnant women. (Library of Congress)

Kelsey's persistence for full testing of the drug prior to approval was vindicated when the epidemic in Europe occurred with birth defects among newborns to mothers who took Thalidomide. Newborns whose mothers took the drug were born with missing limbs and a variety of other musculoskeletal malformations. Researchers later found that the drug does indeed cross the placental barrier. Kelsey was hailed as a heroine for averting a similar tragedy in the US. In response to public outcry, the Kefauver Harris Amendment was passed unanimously by Congress in 1962. This act required drug manufacturers to provide proof of the effectiveness and safety of their drugs by disclosing accurate information about side effects. The Frances Kelsey Secondary School in Mill Bay, British Columbia, was named after her. Kelsey was given the President's Award for Distinguished Federal Civilian Service by John Kennedy in 1962 and was the second woman to receive such an honor. Despite the horrors of the Thalidomide tragedy, the drug was recently discovered to have effectively relieved pain amongst leprosy patients and inhibits growth of new vessels in certain blood cancers.

The human papillomavirus is a sexually transmitted disease that affects women and may remain in the uterine cervix for years without symptoms. It suddenly strikes and may become the main cause of cervical cancer among women after the age of 30. About 90% of cervical cancer cases are caused by the virus; however, not all women who have the virus will develop cancer. Identifying and treating the viral infection is the most effective way to prevent development of cancer. Another Canadian-American female pathologist is credited for her work in discovering that the human papillomavirus is linked to the development of cervical cancer. She is **Elizabeth Stern** (1915–1980) who received her medical degree in 1939 from the University of Toronto. The following year, she emigrated to the US and enrolled in pathology residency training and became a naturalized US citizen in 1943.

Stern became the Director of Laboratories and Research at the Cancer Detection Center of Los Angeles, California and later a research coordinator at the University of Southern California Medical School. Finally, she joined the UCLA School of Public Health and was promoted to professor of epidemiology. Stern was the first physician to specialize in cytopathology. She focused her research on cervical cancer examining 10,000 women and identifying risk factors connected to the herpes virus HPV. She defined the term 'dysplasia' as the earliest histopathological sign of cervical cancer.

Stern's work paved the way for the development of the Pap smear test which was invented by the Greek-American physician **Georgios Papanikolaou**. This has since become the primary tool for diagnosing dysplasia, as well as providing early treatment and preventing the onset of cervical cancer, thus reducing the disease's mortality rate.

Stern was also the first, in 1973, to prove a link between prolonged use of oral contraceptive pills and cervical dysplasia and cancer. She found that women taking contraceptive pills for seven years had a 6-fold increased risk of developing cervical cancer. These breakthrough studies transformed the disease from a fatal one to a diagnosis which was treatable. This also led to the removal of Enovid from the market—a contraceptive which contained ten times the amount of estrogen than other oral contraceptives. Stern's work drastically reduced cervical cancer mortality, which in the 1950s was the main cause of death for American women. Her studies also revealed that women were more likely to place trust in a female nurse or doctor to perform tests and carry out a gynecological examination. In her later career, she focused on establishing free women's medical clinics in poor communities around Los Angeles County. She herself died of stomach cancer.

Rita Levi-Montalcini (1909–2012) was born in Turin, Italy and grew up to a Jewish family. She graduated with a medical degree in 1936. After the Nazi Occupation in 1947, she accepted a fellowship post at Washington University in Missouri—later being offered an associate research position that she held for 30 years and becoming a professor. As mentioned earlier, her great research contribution to neurobiology is the discovery of the Nerve Growth Factor, a protein that stimulates cell growth, for which she received the Nobel Prize in Physiology or Medicine in 1986. She held dual citizenship in Italy and the US, and eventually moved back to Italy, where in 2001 she was appointed a senator for life for her outstanding contributions to science.

Two female physician immigrants from Europe produced groundbreaking psychiatric research that continues to influence the care of the psychiatric patient even today; below are their stories.

Helene Deutsch (1884–1982) was born to Jewish parents in what was part of the Austrian Empire, today's Poland. During her youth, she identified with and defended socialist ideals. Deutsch studied medicine and psychiatry in Vienna and Munich. In 1916, she was admitted to Sigmond Freud's Wednesday night meetings of the Vienna Psychoanalytic Society. She became a pupil and later assistant to Freud, where she thrived and grew into a bright clinician. In 1925, Helene published *The Psychoanalysis of Women's Sexual Functions*.

In 1935, Deutsch emigrated to Cambridge, Massachusetts, where she settled, maintained a practice, and became a well-regarded psychoanalyst until her death. Her seminars, based on case studies and psychoanalysis, were greatly admired, and attracted many students to her classes. Deutsch focused her work and publications on the psychology of women and Women's sexual functions. In 1944, she published her two-volume work, *The Psychology of Women*. The first dealt with girlhood, puberty, and adolescence; the second dealing with motherhood, including adoptive mothers, unmarried mothers, and stepmothers; she was also concerned with adolescent psychology.

Elisabeth Kübler-Ross (1926–2004) was born somewhat fragile, weighing just two pounds in Zürich, Switzerland, as one of a set of triplets, two of whom were identical. She survived poor health during infancy thanks to her mother's care. She was then hospitalized at age five and had her first brush with death when her roommate died. From an early age, she wanted to become a physician but encountered fierce resistance from her father.

Defying her father, at age 16 during World War II, she left home and performed relief work in several European countries, caring for refugees from war-torn communities and became a peace activist. The image of death remained with her for many years and influenced her thinking about the end of life. Ross fulfilled her destiny when she finally studied medicine at the University of Zurich and graduated in 1957. One year later, she moved to New York and began a psychiatric residency at Manhattan State Hospital.

In 1962, Ross **(Fig 39)** went on to teach at the University of Colorado Medical School and was disturbed by the treatment of the dying. She found nothing in the medical school curriculum at the time that addressed death and dying. She developed interest in the "hopeless patient"—a term that was used to refer to terminally sick patients close to death, with the goal of restoring the patient's

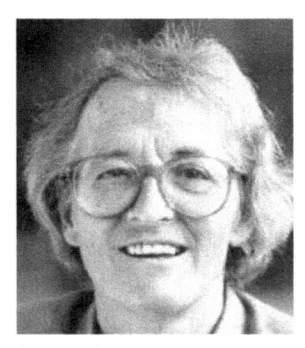

Fig 39. Swiss-American psychiatrist Elisabeth Kübler-Ross introduced the "Kübler-Ross model" with stages of grief and promoted the concept of "Death with Dignity" for the terminally ill. (Wikipedia)

sense of dignity and self-respect. She was also dismayed by the neglect and abuse of mental patients. She decided to dedicate her career to caring for the terminally ill and mentally ill. She developed a program that focused on improving the mental health of her patients.

While in Chicago working as an instructor, she studied psychoanalysis and joined the University of Chicago School of Medicine where she gave weekly live seminars to theology students interviewing terminally ill patients. In the 1970s, she promoted the "Death with Dignity" movement and became a central figure in the hospice care movement. She was a co-founder of the American Holistic Medical Association. She addressed the phenomenon of near-death experiences and reported her interviews with the dying in her internationally best-selling book, *On Death and Dying* (1969) where she proposed the now famous five stages of grief for the terminally ill, also known as the "Kübler-Ross model": denial, anger, bargaining, depression, and acceptance, which became widely accepted. She published over 20 books available in 44 different languages, including *On Children and Dying* (1983).

Ross conducted workshops in many countries on life, death, grief, and AIDS to remove the stigma surrounding this illness. She encountered opposition and resistance, and in 1994, she lost her house and many possessions to a fire suspected to have been set by opponents of her AIDS work. While herself terminally ill, not long before her death, she finished writing her final book, *On Grief and Grieving* (2005), which she wrote with David Kessle.

Ross was the first physician to transfigure the way many look at the terminally ill. She pioneered hospice care, palliative care, bioethics, and near-death research, and was the first to bring terminally ill patients' lives to the public eye. She was named "Woman of the Year" by *Ladies' Home Journal*. Her son, Ken Ross founded the Elisabeth Kübler-Ross Foundation in Scottsdale, Arizona, where she passed away, ready for death and indeed welcoming its arrival.

All these women and others of their time were the driving force behind including women in medical schools and making significant medical advances. By the turn of the 21st century, as many women as men were enrolled in American medical schools—and recently, there were more women than men recorded in medical schools, a triumph long in waiting.

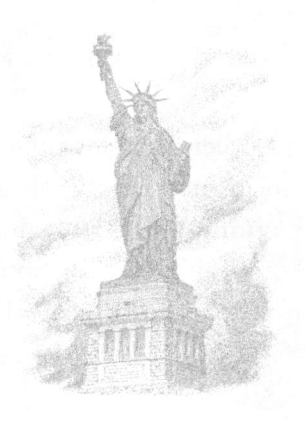

CHAPTER 11

American Healthcare

Medical Malpractice

Hammurabi was the sixth ruler of the Babylonian dynasty, which was named after its capital city, Babylon. He reigned between 1792 and 1750 BCE in Mesopotamia, the cradle of civilization and land of Assyrians and Babylonians, which was located in the Middle East. The Hammurabi's Code of Laws was the first legal document ever used by man and offers a glimpse into ancient Mesopotamian society, its social and judicial order, and the interface between medicine and law. The code is believed to be written by a Sumerian Physician. The laws, which numbered from 1 to 282, are inscribed in ancient Babylonian on a massive, four-ton, eight-foot-tall finger-shaped black stone pillar. At its very top, there is a relief carving of a standing Hammurabi receiving the law. The structure was discovered in 1901 in Susa, Iran and now resides at the Louvre Museum in Paris.

The Code of Hammurabi is one of the longest, most ancient, best organized, and best-preserved legal texts. It has provisions for property, lands, houses, agriculture, commerce, family, marriage, nobility, and slaves. The code is one of the earliest examples of an accused person being considered innocent until proven guilty. The Code also includes harsh punishments, demanding cutting out the guilty party's tongue, hand, breast, eye, or ear. It has a taste of the coarse justice of "an eye for an eye, a tooth for a tooth." It states, "If a man put out the eye of another man, his eye shall also be put out," and, "If he breaks another man's bone, his bone shall also be broken."

The code has information about doctors' fees. For curing a severe wound, the price was ten silver shekels for a gentleman, five shekels for a freedman, and two shekels for a slave. It also includes the earliest malpractice penalties for physicians. It specifies, "If a surgeon performs a major operation on an "awelum" (nobleman), with a lancet and caused the death of this man, they shall cut off his hands." In the case of a death of a slave, only financial restitution was required for the slave owner.

The first recorded case of medical malpractice was Sratton-vs-Swanlond in 1374, when an English woman claimed the surgeon had repaired her mangled hand and promised he could cure her condition, but she was left with a deformity. The judge dismissed the case but set ground rules for future cases, stating that a physician may be held liable, if negligent. The first malpractice case in the US was in 1794, also against a surgeon. The plaintiff claimed the physician promised to operate skillfully but did the opposite and the patient died; in this case, the husband won the case. Abraham Lincoln defended two physicians who treated a man with a broken leg after which he developed a deformity; the case ended in a hung jury.

In the US, medical malpractice suits appeared with increasing regularity from the 1800s, but in the 1960s, claims became pervasive, which increased premiums for medical insurance. Such lawsuits demand time and resources; they can also be emotionally charged for physicians. Physicians often experience those same five stages of grief described by Kübler-Ross: denial, anger, bargaining, depression, and acceptance. Even a jury verdict in favor of a defendant physician can take a heavy toll of personal stress, financial loss, and reputation damage causing discouragement, despair, insomnia, alcohol or drug abuse, and suicide. This has forced some physicians to practice defensive medicine. Despite adopting tort reform measures in some states, the medical malpractice crisis is a leading cause of escalating healthcare costs in the US. Recently, the AMA supported changes in medical malpractice laws.

History of Healthcare

Healthcare is intended to improve people's wellbeing through prevention, diagnosis, and treatment of disease and injury; both physical and mental. Healthcare systems are established to meet these health demands of populations via access and delivery of affordable and good quality service.

Otto von Bismarck (1815-1898) was a Prussian-German statesman who, in 1883, implemented one of the first health insurance programs to provide care to a large segment of workers. Similar systems were later established in England, France, and Sweden. A child welfare movement was initiated by women physicians in the late 1800s after epidemics of childhood diseases and malnutrition, which led to some legislative successes. During the American Civil War, the first personal insurance plan was offered for those traveling by boat and rail. In 1847, Massachusetts Health Insurance of Boston began to offer group health policies. In 1929, a Dallas Texas Group Health Insurance was conceived at Baylor Hospital, where a prepayment plan was developed: teachers paid $6 a year for a guarantee of hospital care at Baylor Hospital; 1000 teachers enrolled. This was the precursor to Blue Cross hospital insurance. In 1933, Blue Cross was established using the Baylor prototype; and in 1939, California Blue Shield began running a similar scheme. 'Medicare is, a government-operated insurance scheme and was established in 1965, with two parts: part A is for hospitalization, and Part B is for doctors' services. This was followed in the same year by 'Medicaid': which is state-operated but financed jointly by the Government and individual States. Medicare provides care to the elderly, whereas Medicaid provides care to children and the poor, including adults. Eligibility for Medicaid is based on family income. Services vary from one state to another; generally, it covers elective in-patient and out-patient services and tests. Escalating healthcare costs and increasing numbers of the poor are jeopardizing the Medicaid system, which has prompted many states to implement reforms. Medicare and Medicaid are nevertheless successful social health programs—which also cover hospice services for the terminally ill.

Hospice Services

Hospices originated during the Crusades in Malta around 1065 and were intended to care for the ill and dying en route to and returning from the Holy Land. In the early 14th century, the order of the Knights Hospitaller of St John of Jerusalem opened the first hospice in Rhodes. Hospices emerged in the 17th century in France; by the mid-19th century, hospices had also developed in the United Kingdom. Modern Hospice care began in England with nurse Dame Cicely Saunders whom herself had chronic health issues, pursued a medical social work degree, and established the first modern hospice in 1967.

Hospice care in the US took root after immigrant psychiatrist **Elisabeth Kubler-Ross** interviewed 500 dying patients and published her book *On Death and Dying* (1969), making a plea for home care as opposed to treatment in an institutional setting and arguing that patients should participate in this decision. While at the University of Chicago's Medical School, Ross began conducting weekly seminars and live interviews with terminally ill patients. In 1969, *Life* magazine brought public awareness to her work. By the 1970s, she had become a champion of the hospice movement in the US and globally. In 1972, she spoke to the US Senate Special Committee on Aging to promote the "Death with Dignity" movement.

In 1988, The American Academy of Hospice and Palliative Medicine was established, headquartered in Chicago, with 250 founding members. Today it has more than 5,400 members, and secured a seat at the AMA House of Delegates. One immigrant-American physician was instrumental in establishing this organization: **Josefina Magno** (1919–2003) was born and raised in the Philippines, where she received a medical degree in 1943 from the University of Santo Tomas. After her husband died of melanoma, she stopped practicing and instead took up the position of Assistant Secretary of Health at an organization in the Philippines. She moved to the Washington area in 1969 and joined George Washington University Hospital. In 1972, she contracted breast cancer, an experience that opened her eyes to the anguish faced by cancer patients and their families. She decided to become an oncologist and pursue hospice work.

Magno went to England and attended hospice courses that combined pain management with psychological and spiritual counseling. In 1976, she established a hospice program at George Washington University and persuaded the Blue Cross-Blue Shield to cover expenses for its subscribers. The following year she established the Hospice of Northern Virginia. In 1980, Magno became the first executive director of the National Hospice Organization. She persuaded Congress to include hospice care as part of Medicare. The challenges Magno faced during the early days of hospice care in the US were substantial, however; a pronounced lack of interest from the medical profession and a general misunderstanding of the concept. In 1980, she established the International Hospice Institute, which became the International Association for Hospice and Palliative Care to train doctors in the US for hospice. Magno is credited with establishing some of the first hospice programs in the US and helped bring the hospice concept into the medical mainstream.

In 1988, she founded the Academy of Hospice Physicians, which evolved into The American Academy of Hospice and Palliative Medicine. Within three years, hospice grew in the US to include 1,200 programs in every state of the country. As of 2022, there were 1,824 hospice and palliative care centers in the US.

A Canadian-born American physician **Gerald Holman** (1929–2012), was instrumental in conceiving the idea with Magno of first establishing the American Academy of Hospice and Palliative Medicine. Holman completed a pediatric residency at the Johns Hopkins Hospital and served on faculty for more than one university, teaching students and physicians. Holman established several hospice programs in Texas, including the Hospice Care of the Southwest, and served on many national hospice boards. His pioneering work for hospice care led the National Boards of Hospice Care to create an award in his honor: the Lifetime Achievement Award for Excellence in Hospice Care. Holman died in Amarillo, Texas.

'Palliative care' refers to pain relief and dealing with the uncomfortable symptoms of severe or chronic illness without treating the disease itself. Palliative care can be end-of-life care, though not necessarily. Patients who benefit from palliative care are those who have suffered strokes, kidney failure, cancer, AIDS, Parkinson's disease, and Alzheimer's.

Hospice care is offered to terminally ill patients with a projected life expectancy of 6 months or less. It focuses on palliation and attending to patients' emotional and spiritual needs at the end of life. Hospice care provides an alternative to therapies focused on life-prolonging measures that may be arduous, involve side effects, or may not align with patients' goals.

In the US, hospices are regulated by government health insurance and offered by private insurance providers, which cover in-patient or home care but do not end after six months. Hospice treatment should be promoted as a reasonable model for end-of-life medicine, but unfortunately, it is still not implemented widely. This is because many hospitals do not have palliative care services and are unfamiliar with their benefits for patients; families are also often reluctant to seek hospice for loved ones.

Fighting terminal cancer is a national struggle that often leads to unexpected emotional suffering; medicine may bring worse side effects than the disease itself and may simply prolong the inevitable. Being alive is also not the same as *living*. Although difficult, physicians should engage in a dialogue with terminally ill people about how many invasive interventions they are prepared to undertake and to discuss their fears, hopes, goals, and what they want for the end of their life.

In his book *Being Mortal* on aging, death, and dying, Atul Gawande called for a change in the entire philosophy of healthcare. He argues against the treatment-at-all-costs model that once prevailed in medicine; rather than ensuring survival, people with serious illnesses should have priorities beyond simply prolonging their lives. He noted that the average cost for a patient to live one year with terminal cancer is $98,000—often involving tests and treatments with painful adverse side effects. About 25% of Medicare spending is delegated to 5% of patients who are in their final year of life, and most of that care will ultimately have little benefit; an obvious example is advanced, incurable cancer. Quality of life should be valued, and many would, in truth, probably prefer not to pay hundreds of thousands of dollars to live a few extra weeks while severely ill.

Outcome Research and Guidelines

In 1900, one in five newborns in the US died before the age of 10. By the mid-1900s, mortality rates had decreased by 50%. Today, however, less than 1 in 100 infants die in their first year of life. Although child mortality from infections was nearly eliminated; among adults, cardiovascular disease, hypertension, and diabetes have become the nation's main killers.

Does this really make much of a difference? President Franklin Roosevelt died of a stroke induced by hypertension. Toward the end of his life, he lost weight, could not concentrate, and experienced severe headaches. There was no treatment for hypertension at the time, and scholars believe that if he had led a healthier life, it would have changed the course of history. A healthy Roosevelt would have convinced Stalin to allow peaceful elections in Europe at the end of WWII, and he would not have allowed him to kill 20 million of his own people. Historians also believe he would have offered support to Mao, thus preventing the Korean War. This is one example of many that illustrate how medical choices can affect our lives in a transformative manner.

In 1905, William Osler recommended absolute bed rest for six weeks as essential in treating heart attacks. We now know this approach is ineffective and, in fact, leads to complications, such as blood clots. Today with better treatments, mortality from heart attacks has significantly declined. The Framingham heart study began in 1948 to look at the cause of heart disease in the 1960s and confirmed hypertension leads to cardiovascular disease. High cholesterol causes heart disease, and high consumption of fat increases blood cholesterol. Medications, albeit with side effects, can control cardiovascular disease, but behavioral factors and lifestyle are important in prevention. Chronic stress predisposes us to depression, gastrointestinal problems, hypertension, and cardiovascular disease. Ultimately, improvements in health have nearly eradicated common infections and chronic diseases, significantly improving life expectancy. We have medical research to thank.

In the 1850s, Florence Nightingale, the English social reformer and founder of modern nursing, studied death during the Crimean War, carefully recording the cause of death—such as wounds, infections, and others. Sixty years later, Ernest Codman, a Boston orthopedic surgeon, noted that hospitals were reporting the number of patients treated, but not how many patients benefited from their treatment, arguing that hospitals should report on the results of treatment obtained at different institutions. Despite these rudimentary attempts at recording treatment outcomes, credit for the first true model for medical outcomes goes to **Avedis Donabedian** (1919-2000), a Palestinian-Lebanese born American immigrant who was a physician and founder of the study of healthcare quality and medical outcomes research. He was also the creator of The Donabedian Model of Care.

Donabedian was born in Beirut, Lebanon, to an Armenian family who had escaped the Armenian genocide for Palestine. His physician father had studied medicine at the American University of Beirut, Lebanon, and established a practice in the Christian town of Ramallah, Palestine—near Jerusalem. This is where Donabedian grew up and received an early education at the Friends' Quaker School, subsequently following in his father's footsteps to study medicine at the American University of Beirut and graduating in 1944. Donabedian returned to Palestine, his home, and worked at the English Mission Hospital in Jerusalem. After the 1948 partition of Palestine, like many Palestinians, he moved to Lebanon. He found himself teaching at his alma mater, the American University in Beirut, where he developed an interest in the quality of health provision and public health. Donabedian then moved to the US, where he studied epidemiology and health services administration at Harvard University, receiving his MPH degree in 1955. He finally settled in Ann Arbor, where the School of Public Health at the University of Michigan recruited him as a professor.

In 1966, Donabedian **(Fig 40)** wrote a landmark article titled "Evaluating the Quality of Medical Care," where he first used the term "outcome" as part of his framework of quality assessment. He listed, summarized, and analyzed the growing literature on health services research. His work explained the need for examining the quality of health provision in terms of structure, process, and outcome. The study brought him immediate fame, and it is still widely cited and read today. In subsequent works, he detailed concepts and methods required to examine fundamental aspects of healthcare. He was an early exponent of systems management in health services and strove to define aspects of quality in health systems and proposed models of measurement in over 100 papers and 11 books, which he published mostly on the issue of quality care. Topics covered include access to healthcare, completeness and accuracy in medical records, observer bias, patient satisfaction, and cultural preferences in healthcare. The summation of his efforts is found in his trilogy, *Explorations in Quality Assessment and Monitoring* (1980-85), a massive work of personal scholarship and thought on every aspect of healthcare provision, suggesting seven pillars of quality: efficacy, efficiency, optimality, acceptability, legitimacy, equity, and cost. Donabedian died of prostate cancer at his home in Ann Arbor, Michigan.

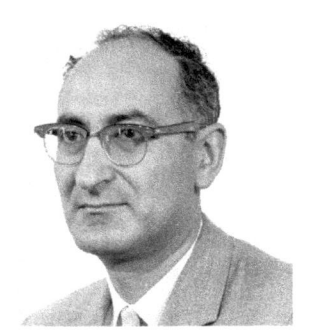

Fig 40. Palestinian-Lebanese born immigrant Avedis Donabedian is credited for introducing the quality care model the first true model for medical outcomes or The Donabedian Model of Care. (Healthcare Market Review).

There are still uncertainties in medicine about the cause and cure of certain diseases. Medicine is a science but also an art. A patient with one disease who consults ten physicians may be diagnosed with three different conditions, and when these physicians agree on a certain diagnosis, they may then suggest five different treatments. This is because decision-making relies on a doctor's training, continuing education, personal experience, biases, and interpretation of conflicting findings in the medical literature. After Donabedian's work, outcome research took up roots in the US in the 1970s and is now conducted to consider what treatments work best. Now, outcome research is standard and is used for outcome management and Clinical Practice Guidelines, which are based on an examination of current knowledge within the paradigm of evidence-based medicine.

Medical guidelines began to be created by federal agencies in the 1990s with the goal of reducing medical costs. Physicians still hold the greatest stake in this matter, though their medical organizations and specialties, upon recommendation from AMA, create independent guidelines for the purposes of efficiency. Some studies show guidelines have decreased the number of procedures and thus decreased cost; for example, it was established that not administering routine pre-operation antibiotics for minor procedures does not increase the likelihood of wound infection.

Guidelines quickly gained political support, and some states moved to ensure guidelines were followed as a defense against malpractice. Guidelines are here to stay, but some doctors are wary of them as they risk becoming a model of "cookbook medicine." Although helpful in decision-making, they are not etched in stone and must be viewed as a strategy rather than dogma; doctors' experience plays a crucial role in decision-making. Good judgment comes from experience, and experience comes from a combination of textbook medicine and life-long learning, which should always improve quality and reduce cost.

Advocates of guidelines believe they reduce cost and avoid unnecessary procedures but also protect physicians from malpractice litigation and help avoid defensive medicine. Legal scholars debate but offer no definitive answer on whether guidelines do indeed substantially reduce cost and risk. Some courts view a violation of guidelines as intent to harm and influence rewards. Guideline developers, besides investigating the evidence for outcomes, should always be mindful of benefits and costs, though not fixated on them.

Problems with American Healthcare

The US medical care system is in crisis, and healthcare itself is a sick and broken system. The problems are too varied to be resolved easily. Most scholars agree that three major challenges for US healthcare are, however: high cost, poor quality, and limited access.

The cost is high for both the patient and the nation. In the 1980s, healthcare costs began to skyrocket, and the cost of health insurance for the average person became unaffordable for many Americans. In 2023, the average annual health insurance premium for an individual at 40 years of age is $6,000—and over $11,600 for anyone aged 60 or above. This is more than what an average person spends on their car, computer, and television combined. The days of $20 copayments and $500 deductibles are long gone. Medicare annual premiums are not cheap either; they depend on the plan (A, B, C, or D) and the individual's income. Plan B for someone on a low-income costs $1,968; and for a high-income person, it is $6,720. According to the CMS, National health expenditure has grown to $4.3 trillion in 2021—or $12,914 per person—and accounts for 18.3% of our Gross Domestic Product.

Quality of care rarely matches cost for most patients. Americans face enormous bills for mediocre and substandard care. Although the US is viewed as having the best healthcare in the world, it is severely lagging in mortality rates from treatable and preventable diseases. Despite its notoriously high cost, health care also has serious quality problems. Having "good" health insurance does not guarantee receiving good care. Many continue to die from poor care and mistakes. Most medical harm comes from system errors than human errors. The Institute of Medicine has found a chasm, rather than a gap, between the healthcare quality Americans are receiving and what they should receive; they subsequently made an urgent call for fundamental change to close the quality gap. The 1999 Institute of Medicine report *To Err is Human: Building a Safer Health System* broke the silence about medical errors, plainly stating that 98,000 Americans die in hospitals annually because of preventable mistakes, poor technique, or inattention to details. This observation jolted health reformers and forced them to usher in a new era of quality improvement.

Access to care is the third major problem of American healthcare. Because of the high cost, many have lost access to health insurance—the aging baby boomers are driving a severe cost escalation. Adding preexisting conditions to the lists of those covered by insurance companies has made healthcare access to patients all the more difficult. In 2021, nearly 30 million Americans were uninsured, a decrease from a decade ago because the Affordable Care Act, but remains high. Hospital emergency departments have become sanctuaries for the uninsured seeking basic care. A 2022 survey found that 43% of working-age adults were inadequately insured. In one study, the US ranked last among 11 industrialized countries on measures of health system quality, efficiency, access to care, equity, and healthy lives.

These challenges for US health care are frustrating for both patients and physicians. Patients face bureaucracy from hospitals when seeking simple X-rays, EKGs, or blood tests. They stand in line at registration desks and fill in numerous information forms, while payments are often demanded in advance. Patients wait too long for approval from their insurance for tests and surgical procedures.

American doctors treat diseases ranging from colds to cancer and face escalating quantities of paperwork and regulations. They see more patients in emergency settings unable to pay for their care. Insurance companies often deny doctors payments. Doctors are incurring greater expenditure and benefitting from lower rates of reimbursement. Physicians are constantly haunted by the threat of malpractice lawsuits. We have high malpractice insurance premiums. In 2022, depending on the specialty, surgeons pay $30,000 to $50,000 a year for malpractice premiums. The costs of running a medical practice have also drastically increased since the introduction of Electronic Medical Records, which require constant expensive IT support. Electronic Medical Records do offer information exchange, but they also instigate frustrating barriers. We so often face mistrust from our patients because of their insurance companies. Physicians are subject to reviews from private and managed care insurers—HMOs and PPOs—who monitor care provided by doctors and sometimes refuse to approve tests or procedures, which places limitations on what doctors can do for their patients. Practicing physicians have to learn and navigate these constantly changing delivery regulations and contend with punitive federal laws.

Enormous problems face both patients and doctors from public and managed care insurers. Medicare reimbursement reductions are worsening. Blue Cross and Blue Shield remains the most popular and widely used private health insurance company. Nowadays, managed care insurers see doctors as providers, and patients as customers. Insurance companies are front and center of an initiative that is damaging the reputation of the healthcare industry. They are the prime culprit for the changing relationship between hospital and physician, and physician and patient. They are constantly changing reimbursement rules and bundling services. They are becoming increasingly brazen about "overpayment recovery"—requesting refunds of payments they made to physicians up to two years ago for services they have already approved. The excuse is often for not including the correct modifier or ICD 10 code. There is no reason for insurers to take four to six months to pay a claim other than the fluctuating value of that money; the longer they take to pay a claim, the higher their profits. Physicians are increasingly frustrated by the denial of appeals, with specific private insurers regularly abusing doctors with impunity. Their denials of care for patients and doctors are escalating. Private insurers also impose restrictions on what services patients can receive and what doctors can offer. Unfortunately, US politicians are contributing to this, which is now becoming increasingly politicized and polarized. Many are influenced by donations they receive from lobbyists and industry, leading to slack regulation by the government, allowing insurers a free hand in canceling insurance, denying claims and out-of-pocket expenses, including deductibles, co-pays, and preexisting conditions. These challenges are causing burnout for physicians and driving some physicians to work at hospitals or else retire early.

Sometimes, patients and physicians are part of the problem. America is rated 35 out of 169 countries in terms of overall citizens' health. About 60% of Americans live with at least one chronic health condition; many of these are preventable through a simple lifestyle modification. Low health literacy means poor outcomes. Some patients go to physicians requesting treatment and expect that an employer or the government will pay the bill without knowing there is a substantial out-of-pocket expense that will be incurred. Knowledge of this cost may deter the patient from consenting to an expensive test or any surgery where there may be other alternatives. Physicians are supposed to give the patients treatment options because when doctors recommend surgery, the patient relies entirely on the physician's judgment and rarely asks for no-frills cost reduction, as they would when buying a car.

In a survey from Johns Hopkins Hospital of 2100 physicians, 20% of overall medical care was reported to be unnecessary—mostly driven by a fear of malpractice. Overtreatment does exist, mainly as a form of defensive medicine, but it also depends on the physician's ownership of equipment or facility partnership, as well as patient demands.

Managed care was plausible simple idea by having primary care physicians ensure patients are not getting too much or too little care, but it strayed path and to cut cost HMO and PPO planners negotiated aggressively with physicians and limited access of patients' necessary care by specialists. To cut cost managed care insurers sometimes reluctantly approve tests and procedures, and subject physicians to utilization review. Doctors' staff waits long while calling an 800 number to approve treatments that sometimes do not come.

Managed care can decrease cost on expenses but offers less access to quality care; it is broadly disliked by patients and physicians because insurers demand discounts from physicians, pay doctors less, and keep more money for themselves, while patients receive less of their much-needed care. HMO and PPO are not consumer-focused models because they limit patients' choice of doctors. Managed care plans make a profit from their healthy beneficiaries. Managed care also places restrictions on hospitals by limiting a patient's stay and reducing hospitalization time. There are instances of morbidity and even death where treatments were denied by managed care—it is quickly becoming 'mangled care.'

Remedies and Reform of our Healthcare

Surveys in the 1990s show that 90% of Americans believe that the American healthcare system is dysfunctional and fundamental change is needed. Patients, employers, employees, physicians, and hospitals are unsatisfied with the current situation. The US has the highest spending and highest rate of dissatisfaction with healthcare, and Americans are not getting better care than other countries. Health reform strategies are, however, decreasing cost, enhancing quality, and improving access. This solution is not simple but is attainable. Health reform in the US has proven challenging in the past. The problem is a lack of political will among politicians of all stripes.

The value-based healthcare concept, which was introduced by Michael Porter and Elizabeth Teisberg (2006), is a framework for restructuring healthcare systems that gained traction with the goal of improving value for patients. It measures health outcomes per unit of cost, and the system emphasizes restructuring and transitioning toward bundled payments, performance-based payments, and capitation for quality. Advocates for value-based care believe that the fee-for-service system, which emphasizes volume, will be completely replaced by payment for value. Government began gradually implementing this system, and a substantial portion of Medicare physicians are now participating in at least one value-based model. Wellness and prevention are positive aspects of value-based care, along with cutting costs. Value-based healthcare groups may, however, delay the referral of patients to specialists and prioritize cost over quality. The system lacks transparency in data collection and places a burden on physicians who take on responsibility for wellness, a convoluted system of payment, and potential penalties. Most importantly, the system does not address one of the three main problems of healthcare: access.

For American health system reform to materialize, all aspects of the problem must be addressed. Past solutions targeted some but not all facets of the problem. As such, reformers' efforts failed at every attempt to reform the system. Certain reforms have been made over the past 20 years and have had some success but still fallen short. We need an all-hands-on-deck approach, and all stakeholders must be part of the solution: patients, physicians, hospitals, payers, politicians, society, and government all have responsibility.

Patients' responsibility

A Dutch-born immigrant physician **Isidore Snapper**, who was discussed earlier, was an early advocate of prevention. He conducted research published in 1941 on heart disease and emphasized the importance of prevention of the heart disease by consuming plant foods and increasing one's intake of linolenic acid, which belongs to the omega-3 fatty acids group.

Risky behavior on the part of the patient is a thorny issue, but patients should have skin in the game and bear responsibility for unhealthy behaviors. Obesity has an adverse impact on health and the malevolent causes of chronic conditions: diabetes, hypertension, and heart disease. Obese patients who adopt a healthy lifestyle by losing weight should pay less for their insurance premiums. Engaging in wellness programs and healthy lifestyles involving regular exercise and avoiding smoking, drugs, and alcohol will cost society much less in the long run. Two weeks' stay in Neonatal Intensive Care Unit for a premature Low birth weight newborn may cost $200,000.00. If mothers do not smoke during pregnancy this money is saved. Economic stability, education, social life, environment, and quality of healthcare are the five social determinants of health that influence an individual or group.

Physicians' responsibility

Unfortunately, some doctors and hospitals are over-implementing tests for profit, either due to meager reimbursement from insurers or patient demand for tests that may not serve any purpose. It has been suggested that doctor ownership of specialist equipment, such as MRI and CT scanners or ultrasound, is linked to an increase in their use. When reimbursements improve, doctors will—and should—distance themselves from investing in these gadgets and disclose any conflict of interest.

The concern that litigation will force doctors to practice defensive medicine should be abandoned. Doctors simply must not order unnecessary tests. Routine preoperative chest X-rays, laboratory tests, and antibiotics should always be avoided where possible. A well-informed patient is a cooperative patient and less likely to have adverse treatment outcomes. Explaining a condition to a patient is time well spent; a patient who admires his doctor will never seek legal action against that doctor if complications do develop. Lithuanian-American cardiologist **Bernard Lown** in his book *The Lost Art of Healing: Practicing Compassion in Medicine* (1999) articulated the importance of empathy in medicine. He stated that the real crisis in medicine today is the loss of the fundamental human relationship between doctor and patient—true healers should use listening and sympathetic language to cultivate a relationship of trust.

Physicians have a social contract with broader society and should volunteer medical care and offer medical charity. They must have zero tolerance for a lack of ethics and professionalism, and adopt evidence-based medicine. Independent medical research must be devoid of any conflict of interest in order to provide truthful information. Commercially sponsored research by pharmaceutical companies and medical machinery manufacturers is often biased and driven by profit.

Hospitals' responsibility

Administrators must espouse practices that strengthen ties between hospital and customer to promote patient and physician satisfaction. They should focus on achieving quality outcomes. Patient-focused care encourages hospitals away from a fragmented, bureaucratic model toward a patient-centered paradigm. Hospitals should be customer-oriented. The old power hierarchy pyramid with trustees and administrators at the top and with employees and customers at the bottom must be turned upside down to put customers first.

Hospitals need to curtail bureaucracy in medicine. Managers should minimize patient movements, increase time spent on care, reduce the number of employees with whom the patient interacts, simplify paperwork, and adapt the milieu to patient needs. Besides patient care, hospitals, whether for-profit or not-for-profit, should reach out to the community and provide services like free clinics, screening for chronic illness, providing vaccinations and information about disease epidemics, sponsor food banks, and address the opioid epidemic through drug take-back programs.

Hospitalizations are expensive. Any means for lowering in-patient costs should be sought by administrators in partnership with physicians. Hospital supervisors must eliminate the massive daily waste in the operating rooms, consider recycling, and make smarter purchasing decisions.

Payers' responsibility

Until a better healthcare system is adopted, payers or private insurance companies should reduce out-of-pocket expenses to patients. They should make their contracts with physicians user-friendly. They should offer incentives for doctors to perform conservative procedures and temper their policies to avoid delaying patient care or denying payments to physicians. Patients should have an unrestricted choice of their provider and unrestricted choice of their health plan.

Politicians' responsibility
Financial relationships between politicians and professional lobbyists and industry must follow ethical guidelines in order to avoid any conflict of interest and not influence politicians' decisions. Politicians, policymakers, and healthcare leaders should introduce legislation to help in reporting healthcare outcomes, encourage private and public sector initiatives that reform healthcare, and overhaul anti-trust and malpractice laws. They should continue making laws rendering medications from big Pharma affordable not only to Medicare recipients but to all consumers through a lower prescription cost. They should have the political will to make agreements among themselves and not use healthcare as a political football.

Society's responsibility
Society should embrace preventive care for acute and chronic diseases, ensuring early diagnoses and preemptive control of disease, which saves lives and money. It is estimated that one-half of all lifetime health expenditures are consumed in the last six months of patients' lives. Society should reconsider notions of end-of-life care and implement hospice care for the terminally ill. Operating on elderly, terminally ill patients will not cure the disease or significantly change life expectancy.

Government responsibility
After twenty years of slumber, Rip van Winkle has seen some draconian changes in American politics. Nothing has really changed over the past 100 years; attempts at reforming healthcare to make it universal came close to fruition on several occasions, only to retreat at every instance. It is time for those ideological divisions, which are the obstacles to universal healthcare, to be overcome. During the Progressive Era, President Theodore Roosevelt unsuccessfully supported health insurance because he believed that no country could be strong when its people were sick and poor. Reform was also proposed for healthcare in

1918, but considered a bad idea. During the Roosevelt tenure, two attempts were made in 1935 and in 1939 (the Wagner Act) to push for national health insurance, but neither succeeded. In 1945, President Truman introduced the New Deal with a National Health Plan, but this was also overturned. President Clinton proposed major health reform in 1992, but it was defeated. Republican Congress attempted in 1995 to overhaul Medicare and Medicaid but was also unable to do so.

In 1920, the AMA denounced national health care, fearing government interference in physician-patient relationships. Critics of universal healthcare are concerned about long waiting times; a decrease in the quality of healthcare; requirements for healthy people to pay for the medical care of the sick; rising healthcare expenditures due to the high cost of implementation; and unnecessary government overreach into the lives of Americans and the industry.

Most studies however, suggest that a single-payer universal healthcare system would benefit the US. A 2020 study published in The Lancet proposed a Medicare for All Act would save 68,000 lives and $450 billion in national healthcare expenditure annually. A 2022 study published in the *PNAS* found that a single-payer universal healthcare system would have saved 212,000 lives and averted over $100 billion in medical costs during the COVID-19 pandemic.

Universal health care is a broad concept with one common denominator for all its various programs, whereas government action is aimed at extending access as widely as possible. As of 2022, there are 32 foreign countries with universal health care for their citizens. Many of these countries also have an active social services network in place that addresses the "whole person" before and after encounters with providers, something we struggle with in the US.

Universal healthcare allows everyone—especially the poor—to have health insurance covering their basic health. There are many possibilities for universal health care, but let's consider one. The government now offers health insurance programs that can be a model for universal care. This insurance covers the US president, members of Congress, and government employees, all the way down to postal workers. The government receives bids from insurance companies and contracts with one. Government organizes the system, but it is not the insurer. To qualify for the contract, the insurance company offers the same rate for all and cannot deny those with a preexisting condition or care for any reason. The Medicare system works somehow in a similar manner. Such a system can be expanded to cover all who want it for a fee. Another alternative is for a single-payer system, where government increases income taxes and eliminates existing private insurance, like the Canadian system.

It is inconceivable that in a country as rich as the US, not everyone can receive care. The cost of covering everyone will always pay off because the general population will be healthier and requires less care. Some suggest that the amount we spend on healthcare already is sufficient to provide universal coverage. Universal coverage is not necessarily government coverage. The word national is wrongly associated with a total government takeover. National health care means national coverage, not necessarily government control. Also, some politicians use the word "social medicine" to intimidate that communism is taking over! In fact, Medicare, Medicaid, and social security are all successful public social programs.

Since the Flexner report, medical schools have been teaching students two sciences: basic and clinical medicine. Recently, the AMA created an initiative to get medical schools to adopt a new science to educate medical students in, namely Health Systems Science. This third pillar of medical education focuses on understanding the complexity of our healthcare system, how physicians deliver care to patients, and how patients receive care through today's convoluted processes. Some issues to be clarified for these medical learners include health disparities, patient access, financing, quality improvement, health policy, advocacy, communication, information technology, and Electronic Medical Records.

Finally, despite these challenges, we should remember that American doctors continue to thrive, providing good care within our system. Foreign-born physicians who have made a home in America have much to be thankful for in terms of opportunities. They also have much to be thanked for in terms of the experiences they have brought to enhance patient care.

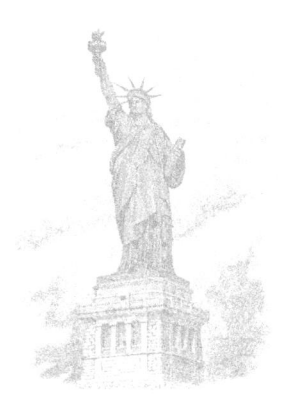

CHAPTER 12

My Medical Journey

My Childhood Encounter with Sickness

My birthplace was Haifa, Palestine—but I grew up, from infancy, in Beirut, Lebanon, and was raised in a modest, traditional, Middle-Eastern family **(Fig 41)**. My DNA analysis shows that 92 percent of my ancestry is Middle Eastern, 6 percent Turkish, and 2 percent Caucasian. The Middle Eastern lineage is from my father, while the Turkish-Caucasian ethnic mixture of my genealogy is from my mother and may be due to the *devshirme* system of the Ottoman Empire, which required conquered Christians from Europe to give up 20 percent of their male children to the state.

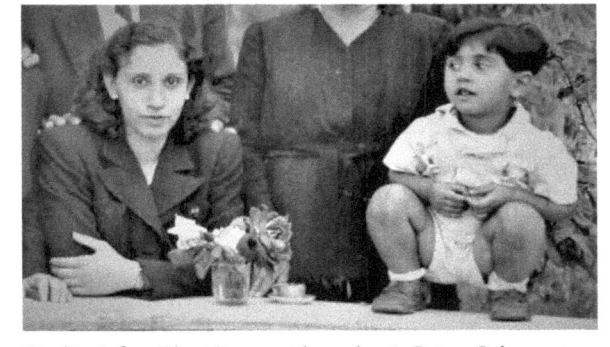

Fig 41. Infant Ghazi Rayan with mother in Beirut, Lebanon in early 1950s.

I became a childhood boy-scout, but was physically fragile. During an overnight campout in the mountains of Lebanon, I nearly fainted from the altitude and exercise (**Fig 42**). When I was six, a pediatrician detected a heart murmur and told my parents that I had a congenital heart disease; he could not predict how long I would live. A child of a family we knew was constantly blue in the face from congenital heart disease and had recently died. "Blue babies" were not a new phenomenon: The surgeon Alfred Blalock and pediatric cardiologist Helen Taussig experimented at Johns Hopkins Hospital with pediatric heart surgery on these children in 1944. Ten years later, the operation had been perfected and performed in the US and Europe, but not in Lebanon. My parents had to accept that I might have a limited life expectancy. I now know that this was nothing more than a benign functional heart murmur that resolves itself spontaneously. As a child, however, my parents always gave me special treatment, and I got away with mischief that otherwise would have earned me a stern reprimand—that is, until they realized I was not quite as near the brink of death as they thought. At that moment, the privilege that I had enjoyed for some time abruptly ended.

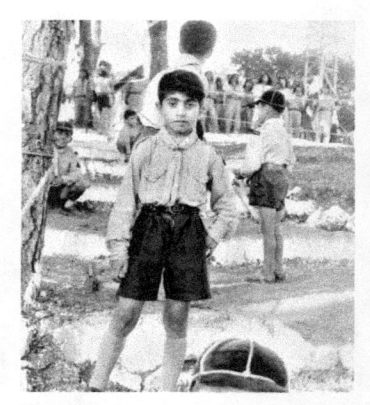

Fig 42. As boy scout in the mountains of Lebanon, 1956.

There were other illnesses, though. My frequent episodes of tonsillitis left a pediatrician concerned I might develop rheumatic fever, which follows streptococcal tonsillitis; he told my parents to consult a surgeon. A week after visiting a surgical clinic, I was lying on an operating table with an imposing French-speaking surgeon ordering a nurse to spray sweet-smelling liquid onto a cloth and force it over my mouth and nose. I was suffocating, terrified, and fighting to get off the table. I was no match for the powerful surgical crew, though. I drifted off into a deep sleep; all I could hear was a loud buzzing and ringing in my ears, along with a ghastly sensation in my head. I remember, during surgery, being partly awake—probably due to the anesthetic wearing off and the surgeon and the nurse shouting at me. Despite its flammability, ether was probably the anesthetic chosen for my surgery. I stayed in the hospital for five days, bleeding from my mouth with pain and the constant sensation of a lump in my throat; I also had difficulty breathing, swallowing, eating, and drinking. It was a traumatic experience, and I kept asking my parents for assurances that I would never have to have this surgery again. Today, of course, tonsillectomy is an outpatient procedure and far less traumatic than my experience.

Sickness also had a presence in my friendship circle. Salah was a childhood friend whom I revered for his ingenuity and adventurous pursuits, especially biking and swimming. His intrepid Tom Sawyer attitude and Huckleberry Finn lifestyle kept me amused. He was sadly diagnosed with advanced colon cancer, and his family was told that surgery could only have cured him if the disease had been discovered early. His passing left me with the shadow cast by that incurable disease and a void in my heart and soul. Colorectal cancer affects older people and can be caused by lifestyle choices or a genetic predisposition. The main risk factors are an unhealthy diet, obesity, smoking, and lack of physical activity. Dietary factors include excess consumption of red and processed meat, as well as alcohol. The condition typically starts as a benign polyp, which slowly becomes malignant. Genetic factors may have been the cause of my childhood friend developing colon cancer.

A family friend of ours became an obstetrician and found work in Germany. While on a visit to Lebanon, he told us stories about the surgeries he performed. Learning what surgeons could do enthralled me. Determined to cure diseases like the one that had taken my friend and not at all deterred by the horrible personal experiences with the surgery I had endured, I decided that this would be my future: surgery!

Later in childhood, I became a photographer taking pictures at weddings and funerals and would help my father with his photography studio before and after school. He had been diagnosed with a gastric ulcer, which was complicated by stomach bleeding—at a time when this complaint had no definitive treatment. Father was offered either an unpredictable life-threatening surgery or a long and wary wait. He declined surgery and was hospitalized for one month as he hovered between life and death, fed intravenous fluids and a liquid diet. The blood transfusion that my father received was only safe and possible thanks to the prior discovery of ABO blood groups in 1901 by the Austrian-American **Karl Landsteiner**. Recent research has shown that peptic ulcers are caused by Helicobacter pylori bacteria and can be cured with a simple course of oral antibiotics. I took a whole month off school to run my father's store and manage its employees while he was recuperating.

My Transition to Medicine

Lebanon was a country plagued by an unsettling series of conflicts that would ultimately lead to a devastating civil war. I was a child with uncertain prospects and little hope of fulfilling my dream of becoming a physician. Yet I dreamed on and studied earnestly, taking English lessons at the American University of Beirut. To maximize my chances of getting into medical school, I enrolled in two grueling undergraduate programs simultaneously in one year in 1967; a science degree in Tripoli, Lebanon, and another liberal arts degree in Cairo, Egypt.

Attending medical school in Lebanon at that time ceased to be an option once conflicts began to close the doors of our medical schools. The romantic drama movie *Doctor Zhivago* was released around that time. The main protagonist was Omar Sharif, a physician whose life was torn apart by the Russian Revolution and subsequent Civil War. Watching that movie only reinforced my determination to pursue medical school outside Lebanon at all costs. I applied to Alexandria

Medical School in Egypt, and miraculously my childhood dream came true when I received a note of acceptance to the most ancient medical school known to man.

I was excited to study in Alexandria. The city was founded by Alexander the Great on conquering the last Egyptian Dynasty, following the death of Cleopatra VII. It was the capital of the Ptolemaic Kingdom (305 BCE-30 BCE) and was also the cultural and intellectual center of the ancient Mediterranean world. The city was home to a succession of Ptolemy rulers, philosophers, and scholars including Euclid, Hypatia, Eratosthenes, and Ibn-Battuta. The ancient medical school of Alexandria was established a full 2300 years ago by Ptolemy II. The ancient medical school of Alexandria was a magnet for many Greek physicians, including Hippocrates, Herophilus, and his younger contemporary Erasistratus, the first known anatomists, as well as Galen of Pergamum.

The first known physician in history was the Egyptian high priest Imhotep. The oldest Egyptian papyrus, known as the Edwin Smith papyrus, describes cases treated by Imhotep. Egyptian medicine dominated global medical knowledge at that time. The Greek historian Herodotus documented Egyptian medicinal practice, and Pliny the Elder wrote enthusiastically of their medical tradition. The ancient Library of Alexandria, built in 290 BCE, once stood tall as a beacon of knowledge. Today, Bibliotheca Alexandria is the 6th largest Francophone library in the world and is built close to where the ancient library once stood. The Library of Congress has the largest shelf space in the world, with over 33 million books housed in three buildings. Bibliotheca Alexandria has a shelf space of 8 million books and a total area of 220,000 square feet. It has four museums, four art galleries for temporary exhibitions, 15 permanent exhibitions, and a planetarium.

To my mind, one of the great attractions of Alexandria Medical School was the English language curriculum it offered, which was modeled on that of Oxford University and unlike any other medical school in the Middle East—which taught in Arabic. Medical schools in Egypt had a 5-year curriculum, which included 2 years' study of gross anatomy and basic sciences, followed by three years of clinical topics.

Egyptian medical schools are state-financed and tuition fees are very low. Under special circumstances, I paid no tuition for the entire five years. Also, because of my high grades in the foundation year, I qualified for a WHO scholarship that covered my daily living expenses.

In the 1960s, we sat on hard wooden chairs or benches in a large auditorium and conference rooms with no heating in winter or air conditioning in the summer. I was nevertheless delighted and grateful for the opportunity. The curriculum was demanding and rigorous, compelling us to lead an ascetic existence and indulge in learning and reading. My professors were great mentors and passionate about teaching. X-rays were a luxury, used sparingly; MRI and CT scans were not yet invented; yet physicians were confident in their diagnosis of many diseases through the time-honored tradition of the physical examination.

My Anatomy Experience

There is a big contrast between the way anatomy is taught in medical schools in the US today and how it was taught in Egyptian schools at that time. Currently, many US anatomy classes involve 6 weeks where students dissect the entire human body. In some schools, the anatomy course is only 3 weeks long, while some spread 24 dissection sessions over a few months. Our anatomy course in Alexandria lasted for 24 consecutive months with sessions twice or three times a week.

Unlike 18th century England, our anatomy class had no shortage of cadavers to dissect. We were organized into groups of 12 students per cadaver. Patients who died in a hospital or in an accident and had no family to claim their bodies immediately became the property of the anatomy department. Individuals typically did not donate their own bodies to medical schools. Some poor people would sell the body of a deceased distant family member to the medical school, however.

The abundance of cadavers and three classic anatomy texts we studied gave us the best opportunity to enhance our knowledge of anatomy. *Gray's Anatomy* text was written by British surgeon Henry Gray and illustrated by Henry Carter—and first published in London in 1858. It today remains the most authoritative standard reference for human anatomy, in the US and globally, and is considered by many physicians as "the bible of anatomy." As a medical student, I studied the 34th edition of *Gray's Anatomy*, published in 1967. My second anatomy text was *Cunningham's Manual of Practical Anatomy* (twelfth edition), which was published in 1958 and originally penned by the Scottish physician Daniel Cunningham. It had three volumes and was a key guide in the dissecting room. My third anatomy book was the fifth edition of *Grant's Atlas of Anatomy* by Canadian-born anatomist JC Boileau Grant, published in 1962. The first edition was illustrated in 1943. To my mind, this atlas was akin to having a cadaver in my own home. In Alexandria, I learned anatomy from a superb group of Egyptian anatomy professors while the authors of these textbooks acted as a second set of distant anatomy teachers.

My first day of dissecting a cadaver, I was memorized with awe. Gazing at the lifeless body was a stark reminder of my own mortality; it was a *Memento Mori*. The corpse was cold and rigid; the joints were stiff; the skin was dark and leathery. Inside, the body organs were bloodless, with brown muscles that had lost all elasticity. The body is partially submerged in formalin liquid and all else is bone dry.

Cadaver dissection is ultimately trespassing upon a sacrosanct body, which has been made into a teaching instrument, thus the cadaver becomes a teacher. It is a sobering reminder that this is what we are all destined to become, no matter how much knowledge, power, status, or wealth one may acquire in life; this is where we are all going

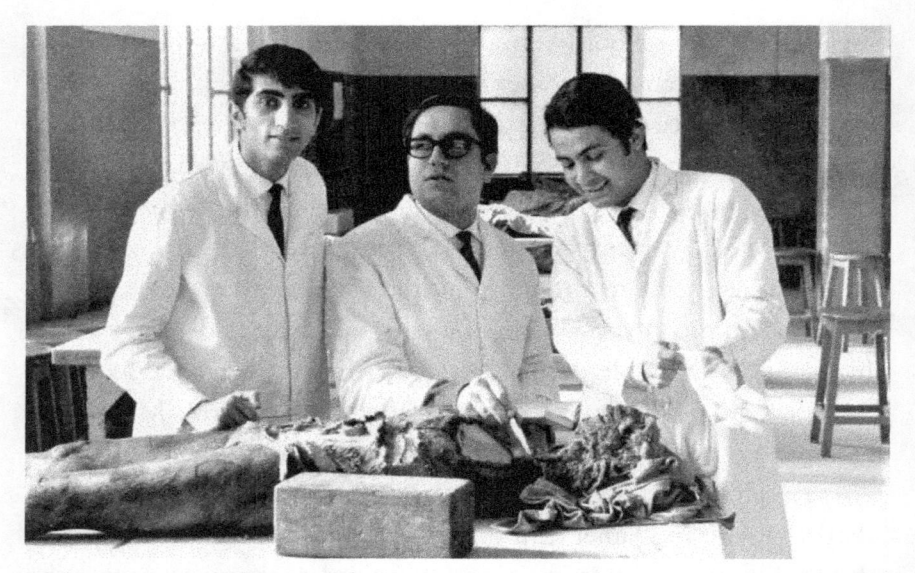

Fig 43. First year medical student (left) during anatomy cadaver dissection with schoolmates in Alexandria University Egypt, 1969.

to end up. It is a stark experience that changes a student forever, but it is the rite of passage.

Several days later, I became inured to the routine of handling a dead corpse. After 2 weeks, the drama of cadaver dissection dissipated, callouses set in and my feeling of angst subsided. The cadaver became a tool of learning, but it was nevertheless fascinating to appreciate that we, the living, were learning from the dead **(Fig 43)**.

An early enthusiasm for gross anatomy was widespread, and most students attended dissection sessions. Weeks later, interest among some students in dissection waned; a few students including myself whose enthusiasm never diminished continued dissecting for the entire two-year course. Dissecting became a routine activity and some students used to dissect without wearing gloves and leave the morgue during lunch break, casually wash their hands, go to the cafeteria for lunch, and return to complete the dissection.

We sometimes encountered unexpected findings inside a cadaver. The intestines often announced the last meal, which often was undigested fava beans. Dark grey lungs replete with black spots would indicate years of smoking. Presence of malignant tumors would reveal the cause of death. Skin and tissue bruising or broken bones showed that accident was the reason for this individual being on the dissecting table. Enlarged liver, spleen, and bladder inferred bilharzia, a common parasitic disease in Egypt that farmers contracted from submerging themselves in the Nile River.

Medical students who had the means would buy an entire human skeleton in good condition for a few Egyptian pounds from the morgue custodian; this practice was not sanctioned by the school. This gave the advantage to those students of mastering bone anatomy. I still own a whole skeleton that I brought with me to the US from Egypt. Before term examinations, some could covertly—for a price—take home an entire cadaver limb to study overnight in preparation for the test.

The two-year anatomy study gave me a formidable basic knowledge needed to become a surgeon. No reading is a substitute for meticulous hands-on cadaver dissection. Medical schools in the US should enhance students' exposure to anatomy with more lab sessions. They rely on voluntary body donations for teaching anatomy, but they are facing a shortage of donations—especially during disease epidemics like COVID—and relying more on visual simulations.

Internship and Beyond

The medical school curriculum was excruciatingly demanding. Before term examination, I used to study most of the day and night with four hours sleep. After five years of a monastic existence, I finally graduated in 1973 with honors, something that only a standing handful of students achieved. I then completed one year of rotating internships; 6 months at Alexandria University Hospitals, and six months in the Ministry of Health Hospitals.

As interns, we had a great deal of autonomy and the most life-changing experience for me during the internship was when the surgical

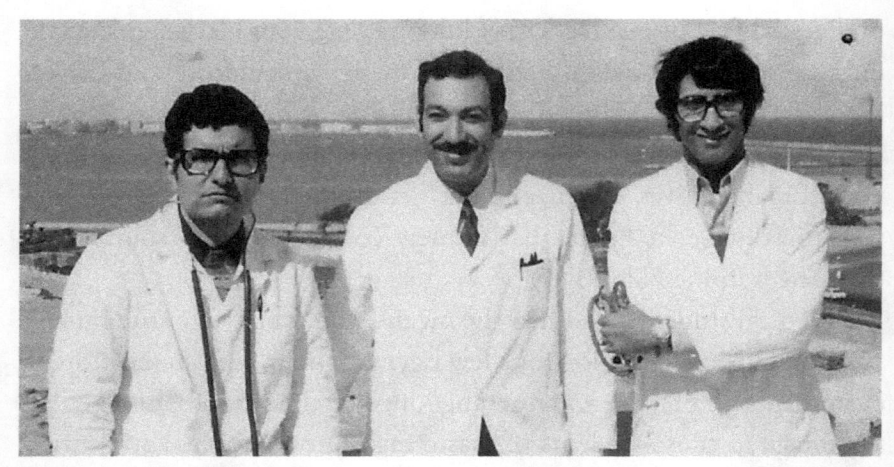

Fig 44. As intern standing (right) with a professor and colleague at the roof of Children Hospital in Alexandria Egypt, Mediterranean Sea in the horizon, 1974.

resident allowed me to do an appendectomy procedure alone. He was too busy to supervise me so a surgical nurse who helped on numerous appendectomies, guided me by telling me what techniques and types of sutures the professors use on their private patients. The surgery went well, and the patient recovered without complications.

On a dermatology rotation, I recall seeing a child with so many head lice crawling in his hair that it seemed gray with crawling creatures. On orthopedic rotation, I would make rounds on a ward in Nariman Bone Hospital where several patients were lying in bed, some in whole body casts, which was the customary treatment for tuberculosis infection of the spine. These patients stayed in hospital beds for several weeks. During my oral examination, the orthopedic professor was truly impressed by my answers; he gave me an A grade and asked if I was planning to become an orthopedic surgeon. Whether my enthusiasm for orthopedics is what earned me the grade, or the grade was the compass that directed me toward the specialty is open to debate. On obstetrics rotation, I delivered dozens of babies. The delivery suite was a mad house because of the sheer volume of patients; due to the limited number of beds, we often had two pregnant women sitting in the same bed waiting for us inducing labor by breaking their water. To maintain the speed of our care and keep up with the volume of deliveries, episiotomy was used almost routinely. During my internship at the Children's Hospital in Alexandria **(Fig 44)**, I saw some children with congenital anomalies that further sparked my interest in that field.

Egyptians are very congenial, cultured, friendly, and witty people. They have endured great economic hardships over the course of three recent wars with Israel that I have witnessed firsthand: in 1967, when I was in Cairo for my preparatory examination; later came the long war of attrition of 1968 to 1970; then there was the Yom Kippur war of 1973. Despite these adversities, the Egyptians never lost their sense of identity, humor, or fortitude. The seven years I lived in Egypt were one of the most memorable chapters of my professional and social existence. Egypt gave me the medical degree that I had dreamed of, along with all the gravitas, prestige, and status that came with it.

In search of a better post-medical education, I pursued a surgical residency abroad. Lebanon did not have any meaningful surgery education or formal residency training. My brother Dale, who had graduated as a chemical Engineer from Tallahassee University in Florida was by then a naturalized citizen of the US. He encouraged me to seek training in the US and apply for a permanent visa, rather than a temporary stay—which might risk my training being interrupted. The requirements for such a visa were many and stringent. First, I needed an American citizen as a sponsor, which my brother was happy to offer. Second, I had to take and pass an English Language qualifying examination at the American Embassy of Beirut, which I completed. This qualified me to take another more difficult medical examination at the embassy—the ECFMG (Education Commission for Foreign Medical Graduates), for which I studied assiduously while in Egypt. I took the exam and also passed. Taking an unfamiliar multiple-choice examination and learning about many medical conditions mainly encountered in the US was truly challenging.

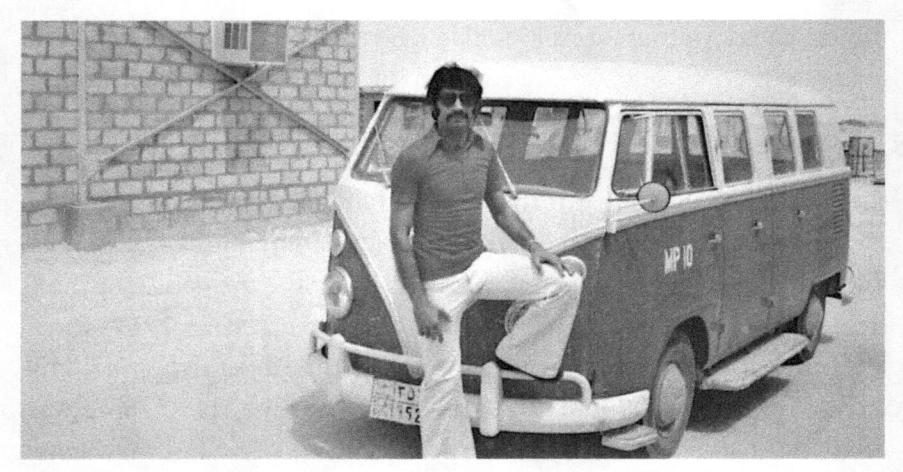

Fig 45. Volkswagen van designated as personal car but used as an ambulance for transporting injured workers to a hospital. Abqaiq Saudi Arabia, early 1975.

While awaiting my entry visa and background check, I worked in Saudi Arabia for an oil refinery subsidiary as the only physician for about 2000 workers, foremen, and engineers. My car was a Volkswagen van that I also used as an ambulance to transport workers with major injuries to a nearby hospital **(Fig 45)**. My clinic was a mobile trailer located within the refinery where the outside average daily temperature was 110 degrees Fahrenheit. On one occasion I saw a worker with a superficial second-degree burn from holding onto a pipe. After three short months, I departed the smothering heat of Saudi Arabia for my promised land. It took one year from the time I applied for the visa until I received it in 1975, the year that marked the beginning of the Lebanese Civil War.

The 4th of July and Struggle for Acceptance

I arrived at JFK airport on the 4th of July in 1975. Contrary to what I had been told, I found New Yorkers to be very friendly. They had parades in the streets that I thought must be in celebration to welcome my arrival to the US!

I stayed temporarily with my brother in Charlotte, North Carolina. That time for me was like a new infancy all over. New faces, new land, and new culture; but there was peace, freedom, and opportunities for exceptional surgical training.

In order for me to obtain a medical license and qualify for residency training, I had to overcome yet another huge obstacle: passing the FLEX (Federation Licensing Examination), a test unmatched in challenge, difficulty and rigor. The test lasted three consecutive days, comprising the three examinations that the US medical students take over four years, and encompasses all knowledge acquired in American medical schools. The material was entirely unlike what I had learned in Egypt, and the process of multiple-choice questions was dissimilar from the essay format I had followed. Despite these barriers, I studied tirelessly and read many textbooks used in American medical schools, finally passing the examination. In all, I took three examinations—two in Lebanon, and the FLEX in North Carolina, each more difficult than the previous exam, before I finally qualified for residency training.

Baltimore Surgical Training

Enrolling in surgical specialty residencies in the US was immeasurably more difficult, even for an American medical graduate. For foreign medical graduates, getting a surgical residency was unthinkable because they have to compete with American graduates for limited vacancies. Getting a residency at Johns Hopkins Hospital was thinkable only to the graduates of the Ivy League American medical schools. For me, engaging particularly in orthopedic surgery was beyond comprehension.

After repeated attempts and interviews, Dr Stan Siegelman, the Director of the Radiology Residency at Johns Hopkins Hospital in Baltimore offered me an externship position—which is akin to residency, but for no accreditation or pay. I joyfully accepted and lived in a dormitory outside the hospital across Broadway Street in a room of about 140 square feet. For four months I studied, while working tirelessly, day after day, with continuous exposure to radiation. For all that relentless work, I was offered a formal residency in radiology, which I declined, because my dream was to become a surgeon. I was accepted for a general surgical internship at the South Baltimore General Hospital, which was affiliated with the University of Maryland.

Then, there was no 80-hour work week restriction for residents as they have today. I was on call every other day, often staying up all night and working in various departments. Today, residents have better working conditions and duty hours than for my generation. One of my rotations was on a cardiopulmonary resuscitation (CPR) team. When called out for an emergency, sometimes several times daily, I had to dispatch to the location and I would perform CPR with combined chest compressions, alternating with mouth-to-mouth inhalation in the patient's frothy oral cavity. Today, CPR is done with artificial ventilation.

During my cardiology rotation, I attended to heart attack victims in the coronary care unit, many of whom did not survive. One of my grim duties was breaking the bad news to the family of the deceased—at the same time, requesting permission and convincing a grieving family to offer consent for the post-mortem of their loved ones, which was required for the teaching program accreditation.

Dr Robert Robinson, the chair of the orthopedic surgery department at Johns Hopkins Hospital **(Fig 46)**, secured an orthopedic residency position for me at the Johns Hopkins-Union Memorial Hospital program with rotations at various hospitals. Crime rates were high in the Johns Hopkins Hospital neighborhood. A medical student, while rotating on our orthopedic service, was shot in the chest during a holdup near the hospital. Fortunately, he was immediately rushed into surgery and survived the ordeal.

While a junior orthopedic resident, my working hours were not much better than when I was an intern. I often took calls every other night and while on call I stayed up most of the night working in the

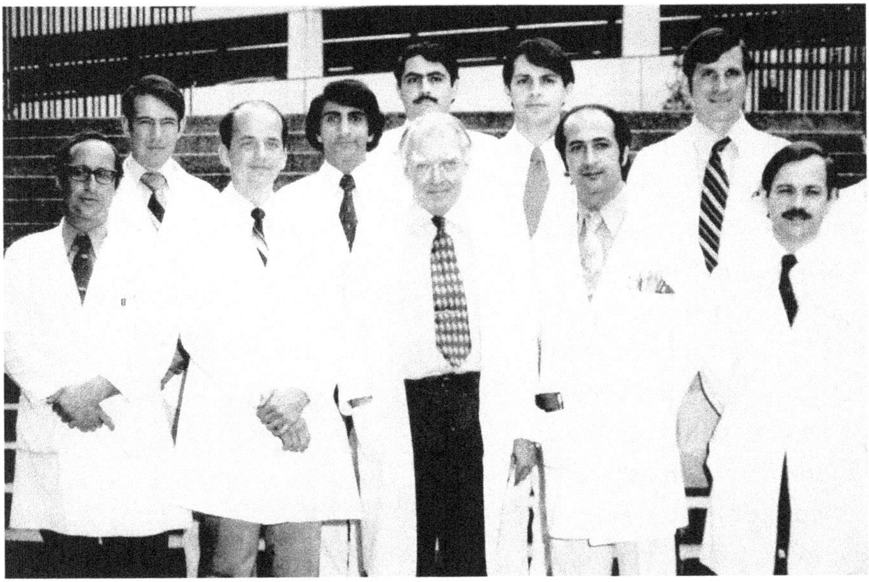

Fig 46. As junior orthopedic resident standing immediately next (left) to Robert Robinson (center) Chairman of the Orthopedic Surgery department and next to Roy Meals at Johns Hopkins Hospital in Baltimore Maryland, 1978

emergency department and operating room. When I was off duty, I stayed in the hospital doing History and Physical examinations late at night on patients who had been admitted for minor surgeries the next day. Patients were admitted to the hospital for two nights—before and after surgery—for simple carpal tunnel release that is done today as outpatient with a local anesthetic. I did menial jobs that nurses or orderlies would do today. I escorted elderly patients who had had a fall at night to the X-ray department and carried out manual evacuation of fecal impactions whose smell remained in my olfactory glands for hours afterward. I set up tractions for fractures, a method no longer used today, and we applied plaster casts, something cast technicians would do today. This while also finding time to read and living on an annual income of $10,000 as an intern with $5,000 extra as a junior resident.

Looking back at those days when I was at Johns Hopkins Hospital pacing around the Halsted ward—on the same floor where William

Halstead himself made his rounds and where William Osler once taught—these thoughts make it all worthwhile **(Fig 47)**. To me, this was the beginning of a career because practicing medicine is not a job, it is a profession. Now, applicants negotiating salaries and signing contracts with the highest bidder may seem to belittle our profession. I was told the more I work, the more I learn; there is some truth to that. Limiting resident hours of work has some benefits, but it is curtailing the educational experience of the learner. Medical education is not training for a job, it is learning skills, inductive reasoning, critical thinking, problem solving, ethics, professionalism, morality, compassion, team-work, interpersonal relations, endurance, and responsibility. We cannot close shop at 5pm and put everything off until the next day. Our trainees today must learn to be physicians because there is no other profession like it. I did survive these tumultuous times of early training. I buried myself in my books and work. As a foreign graduate, I had to work three times harder than my classmates just to be as good as they are.

    I enjoyed working with many of my senior residents and attending surgeons. Many of my attending surgeons were encouraging and inspiring. A small minority were pedantic and patronizing. My laser-focus on learning blinded me to the occasional abusive treatment that I witnessed. While a resident rotating at Children's Hospital in Baltimore, I was fortunate to work with Dr Raymond Curtis, who had a great

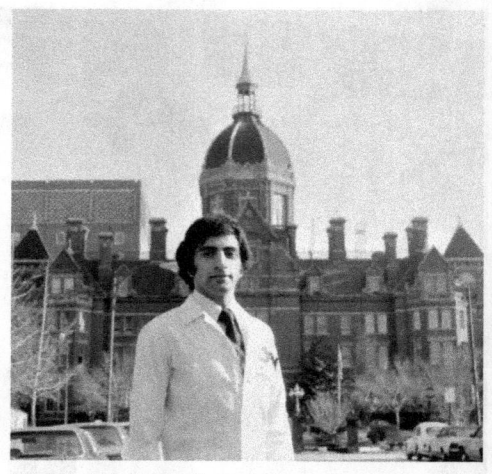

Fig 47. Standing in front of the main entrance to the red brick old domed administration building of Johns Hopkins Hospital. Built in 1889, on 601 North Broadway Street Baltimore Maryland. Photographed 1978.

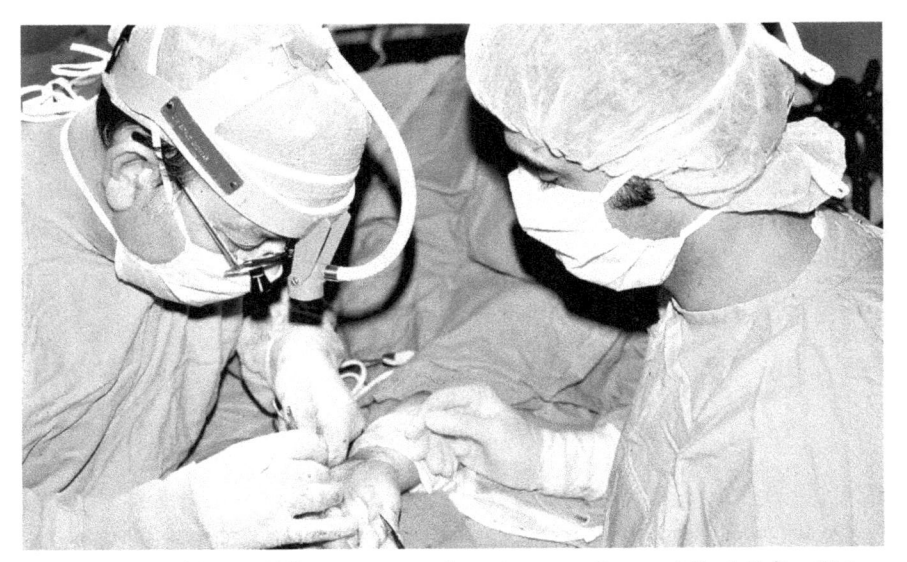

Fig 48. As a Hand Surgery Fellow operating with iconic surgeon Raymond Curtis (left) at Union Memorial Hospital Baltimore Maryland, 1979.

influence on me. Curtis **(Fig 48)** was an iconic hand surgeon and a pupil of Sterling Bunnel, the father of the Hand Surgery specialty. A watershed moment in my professional career came in 1980, when Curtis offered me a Hand Fellowship at Union Memorial Hospital, which I commenced after my residency. Drs Shaw Wilgis, Gaylord Clark, Rick Hansen and Raymond Curtis were the four iconic Hand Surgeons who molded my professional career as an orthopedic hand surgeon—and so it was that I became a second-generation Bunnel pupil.

As a chief orthopedic resident, I had no vacation time, but was able to convince the department chief to give me three workdays off-duty, plus a weekend to travel to Beirut and get married to my future wife, Hoda. I arrived without my luggage, which came the next day. I attended my wedding without a tuxedo to the distant sound of bombing.

My Oklahoma Years
In medical school, I learned about an injury termed the "unhappy triad of O'Donoghue" that afflicts the knee. Don O'Donoghue (1901–1992)

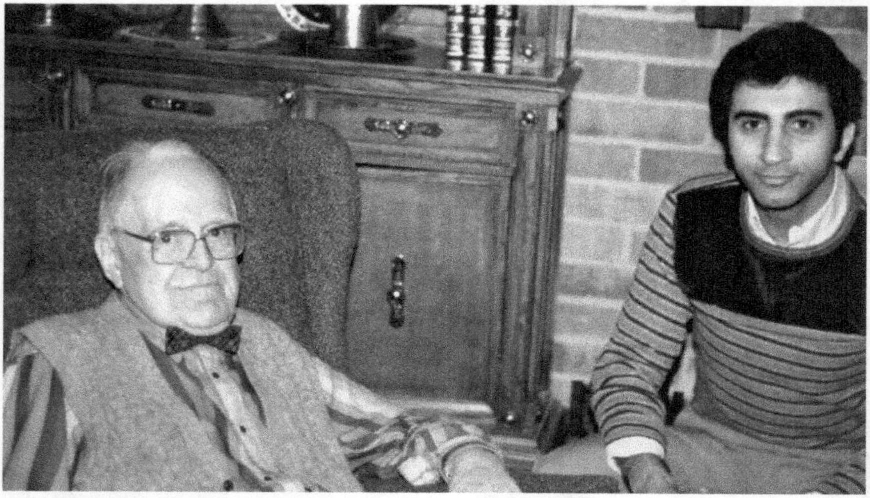

Fig 49. The author (right) with Don O'Donoghue (left) the founder of Orthopedic Sports Medicine subspecialty. Picture taken 1987.

was an orthopedic surgeon who practiced in Oklahoma City. O'Don—as he was affectionately known to colleagues and trainees, described the injury in 1950 which involves tears in various ligaments of the knee. He became the father of a new surgical subspecialty, Sports Medicine, a founder of the American Orthopedic Society for Sports Medicine, and chair of the first Sports Medicine Fellowship in Oklahoma.

While in Egypt, I hoped that one day I would meet this iconic surgeon. As fate would have it, I was unable to return to Lebanon after my residency and fellowship in 1980 because the civil war was still raging. Therefore, I joined the full-time faculty of the orthopedic surgery department of Oklahoma University in Oklahoma City, while Don O'Donoghue was on its faculty—though semiretired. I was fortunate enough to become O'Donoghue's colleague and friend **(Fig 49)**.

At the University Hospital, I was the only hand surgeon in the department treating patients with upper extremity problems, in addition to practicing general orthopedic surgery. I was performing two extreme techniques: fixing pelvic fractures (a very physical operation that requires the use of hammer, saw, plate, and screws) and in the same day, switching gears to then carry out delicate microvascular surgery where nerves and vessels are repaired under a microscope with sutures smaller than a human hair. While at the University, I began giving annual lectures to the first-year medical students about upper limb anatomy and its relation to injury and disease. In my capacity as an adjunct Professor at the Anatomy Department, I constantly emphasized to the medical students, residents, and fellows the importance and need for learning anatomy and the fact that being a good physician necessarily means being a good anatomist, whatever the specialty they seek. There is much to learn from anatomy; I conducted numerous anatomical research studies and learned something new about the human body with every project.

After nearly eight years on full-time faculty, I established an academic private practice based at INTEGRIS Baptist Medical Center in Oklahoma City. Then, in 1992, I established the first and only Oklahoma Hand Surgery Fellowship program in the state, which is affiliated with the Orthopedic Surgery Department of Oklahoma University. The program began training one fellow a year; and in 2001, it expanded by accepting two fellows a year. The hand fellows are surgeons who have completed five years of orthopedic, plastic, or general

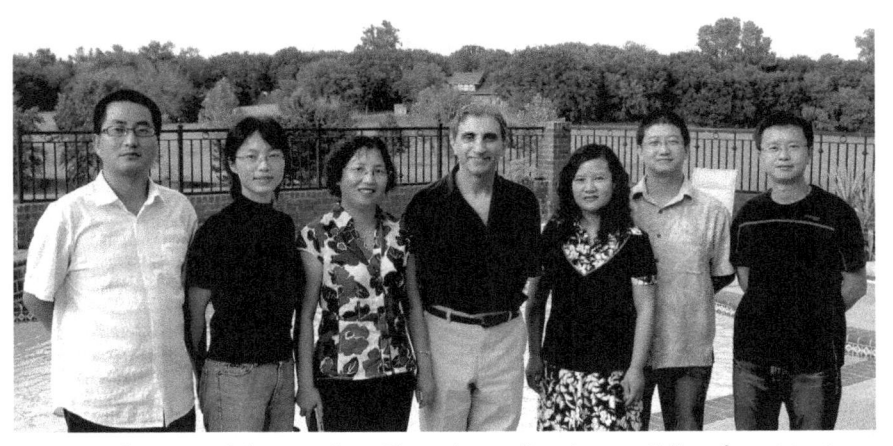

Fig 50. With a group of physicians from China who enroll as observing Fellows for training in various specialties including hand and orthopedic surgery. Oklahoma City, 2008.

surgery training and dedicate a full year during the fellowship to learn the art and science of Hand upper extremity surgery and microsurgery. Since the inception of the program, more than 55 fellows have graduated: 45 clinical physicians and ten internationals, many from China **(Fig 50)**.

American Society for Surgery of the Hand

The American Society for Surgery of the Hand was established with Sterling Bunnell giving its first Presidential address in San Francisco in 1947. Exactly seventy years later, I had the honor of becoming president of the same organization in 2017 and fortuitously gave my presidential address also in San Francisco **(Fig 51)**. The American Society for Surgery of the Hand is the oldest and largest Hand Surgery Society in the world. Today, it has approximately 5500 members. The ASSH

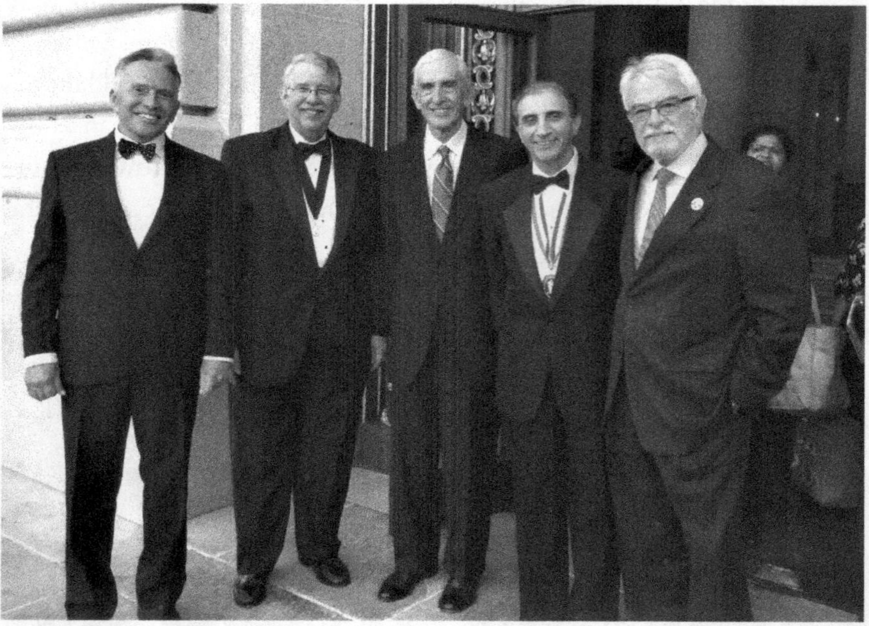

Fig 51. As President of the American Society for Surgery of the Hand, during its annual meeting,. With Past President of the Society David Lichtman (far right), friend Harry Woods Oklahoma lawyer, Andrew Gurman President of the AMA and friend Bruce Day Oklahoma lawyer (far left). San Francisco 2017.

is a global leader and world authority for hand and upper extremity education.

There are two eminent immigrant physicians I had the honor to know and befriend in Oklahoma whose influence on patient care was far-reaching. **Nazih Zuhdi** (1925–2017) and **Elias Srouji** (1921-2015). **Zuhdi** was born in Beirut, Lebanon and earned his medical degree from the American University of Beirut in 1950, prior to moving to the US where he engaged in cardiovascular training. He settled in Oklahoma City in 1957 and became a pioneer cardiovascular surgeon. With other scientists in the 1950s, he revolutionized heart surgery by utilizing hemodilution and autologous priming, which reduces blood transfusion requirements during cardiac surgery. He also worked on improving the heart-lung machine. In 1985, he performed the first heart transplant in Oklahoma. He also performed the first living-donor liver transplant, from father to son, while I helped out with microvascular work. Zuhdi's cardiac care helped innumerable Oklahomans. **Srouji** was born in Nazareth, Palestine and also earned his medical degree at the American University of Beirut in 1944. He returned to Nazareth, where he practiced until 1967, as the only pediatrician in Galilee. He then moved to Lebanon, but the Civil War compelled him to emigrate to the US. He became a professor at the Oklahoma University Health Sciences Center. He trained many pediatricians, and his trainees admired his knowledge and compassion. His book *Cyclamens From Galilee: Memoires of a Physician From Nazareth* (2003) is a fascinating journey into the history of Palestine and the Middle East; it is also an insight into the profound suffering of the people of his birthplace. Elias was a friend with whom I had lunch every Thursday at the Children's Hospital when I was on full-time faculty. My friend Nazih and I also had a ritual of Friday lunches whenever our schedules allowed.

My Story

Although my lineage stretches back to Palestine, Lebanon, and even quite remotely to Turkey, I am loyal to Egypt for the medical education I was offered in Alexandria. My greatest allegiance, however, goes to my adopted homeland of the United States for the opportunity it has provided me to receive the advanced surgical training and academic achievements in teaching and practice. I consider myself part of the human race, a citizen of the world; my religion is medicine, and my sanctuary is a room on the second floor of my house where I can read and write. Education was a gift to me and should be available to all who want it at no or little cost.

My narrative shows that no goal is too high. I am an example of what Thomas Buxton once said: "With ordinary talent and extraordinary perseverance, all things are attainable." Our nation is a cradle of hope and land of opportunity. As a young photographer with limited prospects, a dream, dedication, determination, patience, and resilience, I was taken on a far-reaching transformative journey to becoming an orthopedic surgeon-teacher and president of a prestigious surgical society. The journey I made from photographer to resident to president was not a linear path. I was driven by an ongoing civil war that precluded me from returning to Lebanon. I climbed a long greasy pole to reach my goal. No goal is too high if you climb with care and confidence.

Conclusion

In his 1958 book, *A Nation of Immigrants*, then-Senator John Kennedy discussed what immigrants have done for America and what America has done for its immigrants. The book is a short history of immigration, an analysis of its importance to US history, and an argument for the liberalization of existing immigration laws. Kennedy wrote the book in response to the rising xenophobia and anti-immigrant rhetoric at the time. He stated that, "Immigration policy should be generous; it should be fair; it should be flexible. With such a policy we can turn to the world, and to our own past, with clean hands and a clear conscience."

Later, the legislators heeded Kennedy's crusade; the Immigration and Nationality Act of 1965 was passed by US Congress and signed into law by President Lyndon Johnson. The law abolished the National Origins Formula, a myopic immigration policy instigated in the 1920s. It ended discrimination against Southern and Eastern Europeans, Asians, and non-Western and Northern European ethnic groups from American immigration policy. A man, a book, and a testimony played a key role in passing this law. Oscar Handlin (1915-2011) was the son of Russian-Jewish immigrants who became a professor of history at Harvard University and one of the most prolific and influential historians of the 20th century. Handlin wrote *The Uprooted* (1951), which won him a Pulitzer Prize for History in 1952. The book analyzed the psychology of the newcomers and chronicled the experiences of millions of European immigrants who came to America in the late 19th and early 20th centuries with their own fears, hopes, and experiences. Fourteen years after publishing the book, Handlin testified before congress about the 1920s quota system of immigration and need for reform. In the opening line of the introduction to his book, Handlin wrote: "Once, I thought to write a history of the immigrants in America. Then, I discovered that the immigrants were American history."

Charles Paullin was a contributor to the *Dictionary of American Biography*, edited by Dumas Malone, which comprises 20 volumes and contains 15,000 biographies. John Kennedy quoted Paullin by saying "Of all 18th and 19th century figures, 20 percent of the businessmen, 20 percent of the scholars and scientists, 23 percent of the painters, 24 percent of the engineers, 28 percent of the architects, 29 percent of the clergymen, 46 percent of the musicians and 61 percent of the actors were of foreign birth." Tim Kane, in his book *The Immigrant Superpower: How Brains, Brawn and Bravery Make America Stronger*, argues that preserving robust immigration policy is an essential ingredient for US national security, key to remaining competitive, and a historic part of America's identity as a nation of immigrants.

Some argue that immigration adversely affects the US economy, culture, and global dominance. Illegal immigration may have an adverse impact on the economy. We would do well to remember that in the past, however, immigration has always functioned very much to our economic advantage and that legal immigration should continue to be the foundation of our country's growth. It is impossible to list the many immigrant politicians and financiers who have successfully streamlined the political and financial systems of our early nation, leaving us the global economic powerhouse we enjoy today. Curbing illegal immigration without restricting legal immigration seems a sound policy. America's beauty is in its mosaic of cultures. Embracing diversity and inclusivity has made America the richest superpower on the globe. There is more strength in heterogeneity than homogeneity.

Immigrants took the citizenship oath and later the cadet oath of allegiance, filled the ranks of US military and risked their lives during Revolutionary War, Civil War, WWI, and WWII; they made America stronger than ever on the world stage. We shall never know how many foreign-born soldiers, sailors, and high-ranking military officers traveled thousands of miles by land and sea to offer up their lives in those wars in the name of their ideals.

As immigrants helped America achieve its greatness, immigrant physicians have played a significant but often overlooked role in founding and fostering the medical advances, innovations, and technologies that we enjoy today.

More recent arrivals to these shores have helped meet our shortage of physicians. Due to the scarcity of American doctors in the 1960s, the US invited thousands of international physicians to fill its vacancies. While this policy was intended as a short-term remedy, it became an enduring feature of the US healthcare system.

Concerns for a current or future shortage of medical doctors in the US have been voiced by multiple entities, including the AMA. A study from the Association of American Medical Colleges in 2010 projected a shortage of between 37,800 and 124,000 physicians within the next two decades. In 2010, *Newsweek* published a report that the annual number of American medical graduates seeking primary care has dropped by more than half since 1997.

Physicians in the US are now totaling around a million. In 2019, nearly one quarter of practicing doctors in the US were International Medical Graduates. According to the American Immigration Council, there are more than 247,000 doctors with medical degrees from foreign countries practicing in the US.

In the near future, the country's 75 million baby boomers will enter their elder years. The country's healthcare system will face unparalleled demand for physicians. The demand for foreign-trained physicians will increase as the need for doctors and accessible affordable healthcare continue to grow. About 50% of physicians practicing geriatric medicine and caring for the elderly are currently immigrants. Immigrant physicians are more likely than native-born physicians to meet the need for these less desirable specialty positions; they are also more likely to fill highly skilled positions, such as academic physicians and surgeons. The US shortage of physicians is especially noticeable in rural areas. Foreign-born physicians today disproportionately serve rural and underserved urban communities. They are filling medical shortfalls in disadvantaged areas with the highest poverty rates in the US. Many immigrant-physicians served on the front lines during the fight against the COVID-19 pandemic.

Imagine a world without the explorers, colonists, and immigrants who first set foot on American shores after Columbus' discovery of the New World. Imagine a world where we closed our minds and did not receive knowledge from the outside world. Imagine a world without medical innovations such as: anesthesia or antiseptics; vaccines or antibiotics; tests to diagnose cancers or detect heart arrhythmia; the kidney dialysis machine or heart defibrillator; knowledge of human anatomy and body physiology. This would be our American world without immigrants and their physicians; many medical innovations would simply not have happened—or their discovery would have been delayed. Immigrant physicians have deeply, indelibly, and favorably influenced the American medical landscape. From colonial times to the 21st-century, immigrant doctors have made fundamental contributions in establishing the foundations of America's medical system and influenced American life, culture, and society.

This book is a flying carpet with a journey through the history of medicine and its evolution over millennia. Medicine has evolved with every civilization. Societies perish, but civilizations' triumphs endure. Along the way, we have explored much knowledge about diseases, their history, causes, cure, and prevention. The book highlighted the central role immigrant physicians have played throughout the history of our nation. How immigrant surgeons' efforts during the Revolutionary War saved soldiers' lives and contributed to gaining our country's independence. Civil War immigrant physicians risked their lives on the battlefield caring for soldiers or fighting to save the Union; some were also killed while helping wounded soldiers. Immigrant physicians, during the Rehabilitation era, brought with them European medical knowledge that enhanced patients' care and helped rebuild the country.

Immigrant medical educators disseminated scientific knowledge to students and practitioners through literature, classes, and clinics. Many made novel discoveries in the science of anatomy, while others helped control epidemics. They have come to play a substantial role in US medical research and innovation, something evident in the statistics on immigrant awards and prizewinners in America. Immigrant physicians comprise a substantial number of Nobel laureates and Lasker Award recipients.

Immigrants made innovations in every medical discipline, from anesthesia to antibiotics, from ophthalmology to orthopedics, from radiology to rehabilitation, and from pediatrics to psychiatry. They introduced legislations that enhanced American healthcare, erected hospitals and hospices, and built world-class clinics.

Immigrant physician women joined the suffrage movement advocating for their rights and the betterment of women's medical education while providing medical care to children and the poor in their own communities. Women played no less significant role than their male counterparts in enriching medicine. They led the fight against the prejudice their gender confronted in medical education, and they persevered in gaining the right to matriculate from medical schools. They delivered newborns in obstetric wards, provided quality care to children in nurseries, and offered palliative care to the terminally ill in hospices.

The nonmedical breakthroughs of some immigrant physicians also offered ideas that built some of the nation's historical landmarks and invented practical household items. Their medical modernizations earned them boundless accolades, eponyms, honors, recognitions, and scholarships. One chapter outlined the problems in American healthcare today and alluded to some possible remedies and the positive influence of immigrant physicians on healthcare. The biographies of these medical immigrants should inspire awe and hope; their stories showcase the struggles they endured and the triumphs they achieved; and most importantly, these narratives tell us a great deal about the beneficence of America's early policy of inclusivity.

In the last chapter, I shared my own medical journey as a first-generation immigrant physician. I by no means seek to compare myself with the 140 other immigrant physicians discussed in this book (see list). My intention is rather to share with the reader my own experience of the contrasts which exist in medical education: the anatomy classes I received in Egypt fifty years ago are a world away from the education American medical students are offered today. I also hope to exhibit the differences in healthcare provision in the US forty years ago and what we have today.

Most importantly, I have hoped to highlight the favorable influence of the policy of inclusivity on our country's progress and prosperity. These immigrants' stories are symbolic of what difference they can make, if given opportunities. These immigrants' accounts display the mutual benefits that can be reaped when we embrace diversity. These immigrants' narratives are ultimately an embodiment of everything it means to be American.

References

Preface
- Kaiser-Schatzlein, Robin. The History of New York, Told Through Its Trash.
  The New Yorker, 2021.
- Airhart, Ellen. Rats have been in New York City since the 1700s and they're never leaving. Popular Science, 2017.
- Backus, Paige. Medicine has Scarcely Entered its Threshold: Medicine in the 1700s. American battlefield Trust, 2021.
- Burrows, Edwin and Wallace, Mike. Gotham: A History of New York City to 1898; New York, Oxford University Press, 1999.
- Rayan, Ghazi. Immigrants Who Founded and Fostered an Early Nation, Palmetto; 2021.

Chapter 1: Evolution of Medicine
- Tiner, John. Exploring the History of Medicine, Master Books, 1999.
- Zubir M, Holloway S, and Noor N. Maggot Therapy in Wound Healing: A Systematic Review. Int J Environ Res Public Health, 2020.
- Mukherjee, Siddhartha. The Emperor of All Maladies: A Biography of Cancer, Scribner, New York, 2010.
- Tschanz, David. Pioneer Muslim Physicians. IslamiCity; ARAMCO WORLD, 2016.
- McCarten, James. The Canadian Press Stylebook: A guide for writers and editors, Canadian Press, 2012.
- Asfour A, and Winter J. Whom should we really call a "doctor"? Canadian Medical Association Journal, 2018.

- Teall, Emily. Medicine and Doctoring in Ancient Mesopotamia; Grand Valley Journal of History, 2014.
- Leon-Sanchez A, Cuetter A, Ferrer G. Cervical spine manipulation: an alternative medical procedure with potentially fatal complications. South Med J. 2007.
- Carprieaux M, Michotte A, Van Varenbergh D, Marichal M. Spontaneous bilateral carotid artery dissection following cervical manipulation. Leg Med, 2012.
- Jentzen J, Amatuzio J, Peterson G. Complications of cervical manipulation: a case report of fatal brainstem infarct with review of the mechanisms and predisposing factors. J Forensic Sci. 1987.
- Clifford, Pickover. The medical book: from witch doctors to robot surgeons, Sterling New York, 2012.
- Saving Lives, Buying Time: Economics of Malaria Drugs in an Age of Resistance. National Library of Medicine.
- Medicinal Botany; US Department of Agriculture.

Chapter 2: Anatomical Sciences and Anatomists

- Hutchison, Richard and Rayan, Ghazi. Astley Cooper: His Life and Surgical Contributions. Journal of Hand Surgery, 2011.
- Burch, Druin. Digging Up the Dead: Uncovering the Life and Times of an Extraordinary Surgeon. Vintage Books, United Kingdom, 2008.
- Sappol, Michael. A Traffic of Dead Bodies: Anatomy and Embodied Social Identity in Nineteenth Century America. Princeton University Press. Princeton and Oxford, 2002.
- Schwanz, Mary. A culture of anatomy: The public writings of American Anatomists, 1800-1870. James Madison University, 2013.

- Zaffe, Davide. On The Great Anatomists: A Memory e-book. BMN Modena Italy, 2015.
- Park, Katharine. Secrets of Women: Gender, Generation, and the Origins of Human Dissection. Zone Books; New York, 2010.
- Tubbs S, Shoja M, Loukas M and Agutter. History of Anatomy: An International Perspective 1st Edition Wiley Blackwell, 2019.
- D'Antoni A, Loukas M, Black S. Granville Sharp Pattison (1791-1851): Scottish anatomist and surgeon with a propensity for conflict. Acta Med Hist Adriat. 2015.
- Konstantinos L, Marilita M and Androutsos G. Ammar ibn Ali al-Mawsili and His Innovating Suction Method for the Treatment of Cataract. Surgical Innovations, 2016.
- Bay, Noel Si-Yang and Bay, Boon-Huat: Greek anatomist Herophilus: the father of anatomy. Anat Cell Biol, 2010.

Chapter 3: American Medical Education and Educators
- 200 years of American Medicine 1776-1976. US Department of Health, Education, and Welfare.
- Robley, Dunglison: List of anatomical preparations for UVa, 1825. Founders on line.
- Langer R, Gerster A and Thorek M. contributions to American surgery. J Invest Surg, 2009.
- Thorek, Philip. Anatomy in Surgery. JP Lippincott Philadelphia Taranto, 1962.
- Snapper, Isidore. Meditations on Medicine and Medical Education: Past and Present. New York. London, Grune & Stratton. 1956.
- Duffy, Thomas. The Flexner Report — 100 Years Later Yale J Biol Med. 2011.

Chapter 4: Colonial and Revolutionary War Physicians
- Colonial American Doctors, Gini.
- Fuller, Samuel. Beyond the Pilgrim Story. America's Museum of Pilgrims Possessions.
- Murphy, Francis. The Diary of Edward Taylor. Connecticut Valley Historical Museum, Springfield, 1964.
- Terry, Taylor and Nason, Emma. Rev. Edward Taylor, 1642-1729. Pala Press, 2015.
- The Innovative Career of Surgeon Benjamin Howard. National Museum of Civil War Medicine, 2020.
- *McCulla, Theresa*. Medicine in Colonial North America, Colonial North America at Harvard Library, 2016.

Chapter 5: Civil War Physicians
- Civil War Medicine: An Overview of Medicine. The Ohio State University.
- Civil War Soldiers Record Database. Norwegian American website.
- Bradford, Caroline. The Detmold Knife and the Empty Sleeve: Military Medicine, 2016.
- Biography of Henry Eversman. Effingham County, Illinois; Genealogy and History.
- Dr Henry Eversman: Effingham County, Illinois, Genealogy and History
- Ward, Patricia. Simon Baruch: Rebel in the Ranks of Medicine, 1840-1921. University of Alabama Press, 1994.
- Cabinet Card Photograph of Charles O'Leary, M.D., Civil War Surgeon. Fine Military Americana.
- Thomas Antisell (1817-1893): Young Irelander, Physician, Scientist, Professor, and Veteran of the U.S. Civil War. Fenian Graves: Remembering and Honoring our Patriot Dead.
- Colonel Joseph Thoburn. First West Virginia Infantry.

- Samuel Arthur Jones papers, 1833-1974: Rare Book & Manuscript Library, University of Illinois Library at Urbana-Champaign.
- Jones, Arthur. Thoreau: a Glimpse. Sagwan Prress, 2018.
- Frank Jastrzembski, The Rise and Fall of Brig. Gen. James L. Kiernan. Emerging Civil War, 2018.
- Brigade Surgeon Samuel W. Everett (USA), Geni.
- Doctor & Artist Samuel W. Everett. The Beehive: Massachusetts Historical Society, 1791.
- The Innovative Career of Surgeon Benjamin Howard. National Museum of civil war medicine, 2020.
- Dittmer, Arlis. Death of Doctor Samuel W Everett at Shiloh; Herald Whig, 2014.
- Young, Patrick. Immigrant nurse reports on Civil War hospital organized by Nursing Nuns after Shiloh battle; In Long Island WINS, 2016.

Chapter 6: Antebellum Physicians with Non medical Contributions

- William Thornton (1759-1828), Prints & photographs Reading Room Library of Congress.
- Schneeberg, Norman. Dr William Thornton (1759-1828) a savant of colonial America. J Med Biogr, 2006.
- Dr. William Thornton: First Architect of the Capitol; Architect of the Capitol website
- James Tytler (1745-1804); Editor second edition of 'Encyclopaedia Britannica, National records of Scotland.
- Russell, Meg. Tytler, James [called Balloon Tytler] (1745–1804). Oxford dictionary of National Biographies.
- John Gorrie, M.D. Inventor, Humanitarian, Physician 1803 – 1855. Florida Inventors Hall of Fame.

- Bair, Kevin. Dr John Gorrie "Father of Refrigeration and Air Conditioning"? 2021. kevin@historywithKev.com.
- William Ludwig Detmold : Museum of History, Hall of North and South Americans.
- Simon Baruch: Rebel in the Ranks of Medicine, 1840-1921 Department of History.

Chapter 7: Physicians in the Dawn of Modern Medicine
- Veeder, Borden. Abraham Jacobi. Pediatric Profiles: Reprinted form The Journal of Pediatrics. St Louis. The CV Mosby Company, 1957.
- Lyons, Albert and Pettucelli Joseph. Medicine: An Illustrated History. Abradale Press. Harry N Abrams, Inc., Publishers, New York, 1978.
- Schwartz, David. Physician-Scientists: The Bridge between Medicine and Science. American Journal of Respiratory and Critical Care Medicine. 2012.
- AAAS Resolution: Death Of Dr. James Carroll From Yellow Fever Experimentation. Encyclopedia.com
- Pearce, John. Robert Wartenberg, MD (1887–1956) European Neurology, 2018.
- Leonard George Rowntree (1883–1959): A near-forgotten father of North American nephrology. Athens Medical Society. Archives of Hellenic Medicine. ISSN 11-05-3992.
- The Kidney project; statistics. University of California San Francisco, 2018.
- Viner, Russel. Abraham Jacobi and German Medical Radicalism in Antebellum New York. Bulletin of the History of Medicine, 1998.
- Stephen, Ronald. Adolph H Giesecke, First use of halothane in the United States, (1916-2006). Bull Anesth Hist. 2008.

Chapter 8: Physicians of Specialized Fields

- Schwartz, David. Physician-Scientists: The Bridge between Medicine and Science; American Journal of Respiratory and Critical Care Medicine. 2012.
- Boyed, Joseph. On Shoulder of Giants: Notable Names in Hand Surgery. American Society for Surgery of the Hand, 2002.
- Hernigou, Philippe. Smith–Petersen and early development of hip arthroplasty. Int Orthop, 2014.
- Thompson, Robert. The Smith-Petersen Nail. JAMA, 1967.
- Jay, Swayambunathan, Incidence of Hip Fracture Over 4 Decades in the Framingham Heart Study, JAMA, 2020.
- Gwen, Robbins et al. Ancient Skeletal Evidence for Leprosy in India (2000 B.C.) PLoS One, 2009.
- Caruso, James and Sheehan, Jason. Psychosurgery, ethics, and media: a history of Walter Freeman and the lobotomy. Neurological Focus, 2017.
- Cohn, R. Wladimir Theodore Liberson (1904–1994). Journal of clinical neurophysiology, 1995.
- Adrian Ede Flatt, MD, FRCS: a conversation with the editor. Baylor university Medical center Proceedings, 2000.
- Dobbs M and Khan S. The life and legacy of Ignacio Ponseti. Indian J Orthop, 2010.
- Buckwalter, Joseph. Arthur Steindler: Orthopaedic Scholar, Teacher, and Clinician. Clinical Orthopaedics and Related Research, 2000.

Chapter 9: Award Winning Physicians

- Wargin, Kathy-Jo. Alfred Nobel: The Man Behind the Peace Prize. The Children's Book Council, 2009.
- Morris, James. Politzer: A Life in Politics, Print, and Power. Harper Perennial, 2010.

- River, Charles. Joseph Pulitzer: The Life and Legacy of America's Most Controversial Publisher. CreateSpace, 2018.
- Zannos, Susan. Joseph Pulitzer: And the Story Behind the Pulitzer Prize, 2003.
- Interactions between tumour-viruses and genetic components of the cell. Animalresearch.info 2014

Chapter 10: Women Physicians
- Nelson, Allison. Men and Women in Midwifery. Wonders & Marvels. Vanderbilt University.
- Campbell, Olivia. Women in White Coats: How the First Women Doctors Changed the World of Medicine. Park Row, 2021
- Ehrenreich, Barbara and English, Deirdre. Witches, Midwives, and Nurses: A History of Women Healers. The Feminist Press at CUNY, 2010.
- Minkowski, W. Women Healers of the Middle Ages: Selected Aspects of Their History. American Journal of Public Health, 1992.
- Little, Becky. How Medieval Churches Used Witch Hunts to Gain More Followers. History.com, 2018.

Chapter 11: American Healthcare
- Cutler, David. Your money or your life: strong medicine for Americas healthcare system. Oxford University Press, 2004.
- Vibbert, Spencer. What Works: How Outcomes Research will Change Medical Practice. Whittle Direct Books, 1993.
- Starr, Paul. The logic of health care reform. Penguin Books, 1992.
- Herman H, Weeks, L Kukla S. The financial management of hospitals. Health Administration Pr, 1994.

- Leebov, Wendy and Scott, Gail. Health care mangers in transition. Jossey-Bass, 1991.
- Lathr, Philip. Restructuring Health Care: The Patient-Focused Paradigm 1st Edition. Jossey-Bass, 1993.
- Porter, Michael and Teisberg, Elizabeth. Redefining healthcare; Harvard Business Review Press, 2006.
- Toussaaint, John. Potent Medicine: the collaborative cure for health care. ThedaCare Center, 2012.
- Hupfeld, Stanley. Political malpractice; Yorkshire Publishing, 2012.
- Melhad E, Feinburg W, Swartz H. Money power and health care, Health Administration Pr, 1988.
- Skochelak, Susan et al. Health Systems Science;. AMA Education Consortium
- Josefine Bautista Nagno MD. International Association For Hospice & Palliative Care
- Potyraj, Julie. The Quality of US Healthcare Compared With the World. AJMC, 2016.
- U.S. Health Insurance Industry Analysis Report. National Association of Insurance Commissioners.
- Foreign Countries with Universal Health Care: New York State Department of health, 2022.
- Crossing the Quality Chasm: A New Health System for the 21st Century; Institute of Medicine, 2001.
- Hawley, Pippa. Barriers to Access to Palliative Care: National Library of medicine, 2017.
- Unneeded Medical Care is Common and Driven by Fear of Malpractice, Physician Survey Concludes; Johns Hopkins Medicine, 2017.
- Hay, Joel. Now Is the Time for Transparency in Value-Based Healthcare Decision Modeling. Value in Health; Direct science, 2019.

Chapter 12: My Medical Journey

- Barr, Brook. The Life of Nazih Zuhdi: Uncharted Voyage of a Heart, Oklahoma Heritage Association, 2005.
- Srouji, Elias. Cyclamens From Galilee: Memoirs of a Physician From Nazareth, iUniverse, 2003.
- Woods, H. Day, Bruce. Rayan, Ghazi. Trilogy of Perseverance and Friendship in the Golden Years. Palmetto, 2001.

Conclusion

- Kennedy, John. A Nation of Immigrants. Harper and Row, 1964.
- Handlin, Oscar. The Uprooted: The Epic Story of the Great Migrations That Made the American People. Little Brown and Company, 1973.
- Malone, Dumas. The *Dictionary of American Biography. Charles Scribner Sons*, 1928-1936.
- Kolker, Claudia. The Immigrant Advantage: What We Can Learn from Newcomers to America about Health Happiness and Hope. Free Press, 2013.
- Kane, Tim. The Immigrant Superpower: How Brains, Brawn and Bravery Make America Stronger. Oxford Univesity Press, 2022.
- The Complexities of Physician Supply and Demand: Projections From 2019 to 2034. Association of American Medical Colleges, 2021.
- Miller, Norman. Immigrant physicians: Why are they vital for U.S. healthcare? Medical News Today, 2017.
- Healthcare: New Medical Economy Research Fund.

Other Web Sources
- Wikipedia The Free Encyclopedia
- Library of Congress
- Find a Grave website
- Billion Graves
- American Immigration Council
- Institute for immigration research

List of Immigrant Physicians and Health Professionals

Men Physicians
1. Eugène Hilarian Abadie
2. Anderson Abbott
3. Robert M. Addison
4. Aristides Agramonte
5. Thomas Antisell
6. Oswald Theodore Avery Jr
7. Alfred C Baker
8. Donald Balfour
9. Simon Baruch
10. William R. Blackwood
11. Louis Blenker
12. Mark Blumenthal
13. Geoffrey Bourne
14. Paul Brand
15. Louis Braun
16. James Bryan
17. Abraham Brill
18. Charles Brown-Séquard
19. Francis Noel Burke
20. Thomas Burke
21. Charles Campbell
22. Robert Carrall
23. James Carroll
24. Albert Claude
25. Samuel Clossy
26. Carl Cori

27. Eliot Corday
28. Cadwallader Colden
29. André Frédéric Cournand
30. Richard J. Curran
31. William Ludwig Detmold
32. Alexander De Soto
33. Avedis Donabedian
34. Edward Donnelly
35. William Douglass
36. Renato Dulbecco
37. Robley Dunglison
38. Karl Theodore Dussik
39. Prosper Ellsworth
40. Samuel William Everett
41. Henry Eversman
42. Adrian Flatt
43. Samuel Ferrin
44. Samuel Fuller
45. Arpad Gerster
46. William Goehrig
47. John B. Gorrie
48. Franz M. Groedel
49. Andreas Grüntzig
50. Edward Hand
51. William L Harkness
52. Patrick Heaney
53. Hans Christian Heg
54. Stephen Oliver Himoe
55. Gerald Holman
56. Benjamin Howard
57. Francis (Franz) Huebschmann
58. Charles Huggins

59. William Irvine
60. David Jackson
61. Abraham Jacobi
62. Samuel Arthur Jones
63. Noble Wimberly Jones
64. Eric Kandel
65. Leo Kanner
66. Hamper Kelikian
67. James Lawlor Kiernan
68. Edward Dominicus Kittoe
69. Willem Kolff
70. Karl Koller
71. Karl Landsteiner
72. Charles Frederick Lehlbach
73. Wladimir Liberson
74. Graham Lister
75. Philip Levine
76. Samuel Levine
77. Petter Lindström
78. Fritz Albert Lipmann
79. Otto Loewi
80. Bernard Lown
81. William Worrall Mayo
82. Alexander Maximow
83. James McHenry
84. Colin MacLeod
85. Adolf Meyer
86. William Chester Minor
87. Charles O'Leary
88. William Osler
89. George Palade
90. Daniel Palmer

91. Georgios Papanikolaou
92. Granville Sharp Pattison
93. Peter Pineo
94. Simon Pollak
95. Ignacio Ponseti
96. Keith Porter
97. Leonard Rowntree
98. David Domingo Sabatini
99. Albert Bruce Sabin
100. Béla Schick
101. Ernst Schmidt
102. Édouard Séguin
103. Samuel Sewall
104. Alexander Skene
105. Isidore Snapper
106. Marius Smith-Petersen
107. Elias Srouji
108. Arthur Steindler
109. Ralph Steinman
110. Arthur St Clair
111. Edward Taylor
112. Joseph Thoburn
113. William Thompson
114. Max Thorek
115. Matthew Thornton
116. William Thornton
117. Thomas Tudor Tucker
118. James Tytler
119. William Wagner
120. Robert Wartenberg
121. Fredric Wertham
122. Michael Wigglesworth

123. John Julian Wild
124. Ernst Ludwig Wynder
125. Isachar Zacharie
126. Nazih Zuhdi

Women Physicians
127. Elizabeth Blackwell
128. Gerty Cori
129. Helene Deutsch
130. Francis Kelsey
131. Rita Levi-Montalcini
132. Mary Putnam Jacobi
133. Josefina Magno
134. Gertie Marx
135. Elisabeth Kübler-Ross
136. Rachel Schneerson
137. Anna Howard Shaw
138. Elizabeth Stern
139. Me-Iung Ting
140. Marie Zakrzewska

Immigrant Medical Influencers
1. Elizabeth Blackburn
2. Günter Blobel
3. Lorenz Brentano
4. Mario Capecchi
5. Max Delbrück
6. John Ericsson
7. Enrico Fermi
8. Napoleone Ferrara
9. Michael Grunstein
10. Michael Hall

11. Joseph Keppler
12. Mabel Ping-Hua Lee
13. Choh Hao Li
14. Albert Davis Lasker
15. Fritz Lipman
16. Salvador Luria
17. Catherine MacKenzie
18. Mother Alfred Moses
19. Miguel Ondetti
20. Joseph Pulitzer
21. Oliver Smithies
22. Gunther Stent
23. Thomas Südhof
24. Jack Szostak
25. Alexander Varshavsky
26. Selman Waksman
27. Peter Walter

Other Immigrants
28. Edward Baker
29. Andrew Carnegie
30. Thomas Davidson
31. Christian Detmold
32. William H Harkness
33. Daniel Hough
34. Mary Mallon
35. Gerta Ries
36. Carl Schurz
37. Franz Sigel
38. James Smith
39. George Taylor

GHAZI RAYAN MD

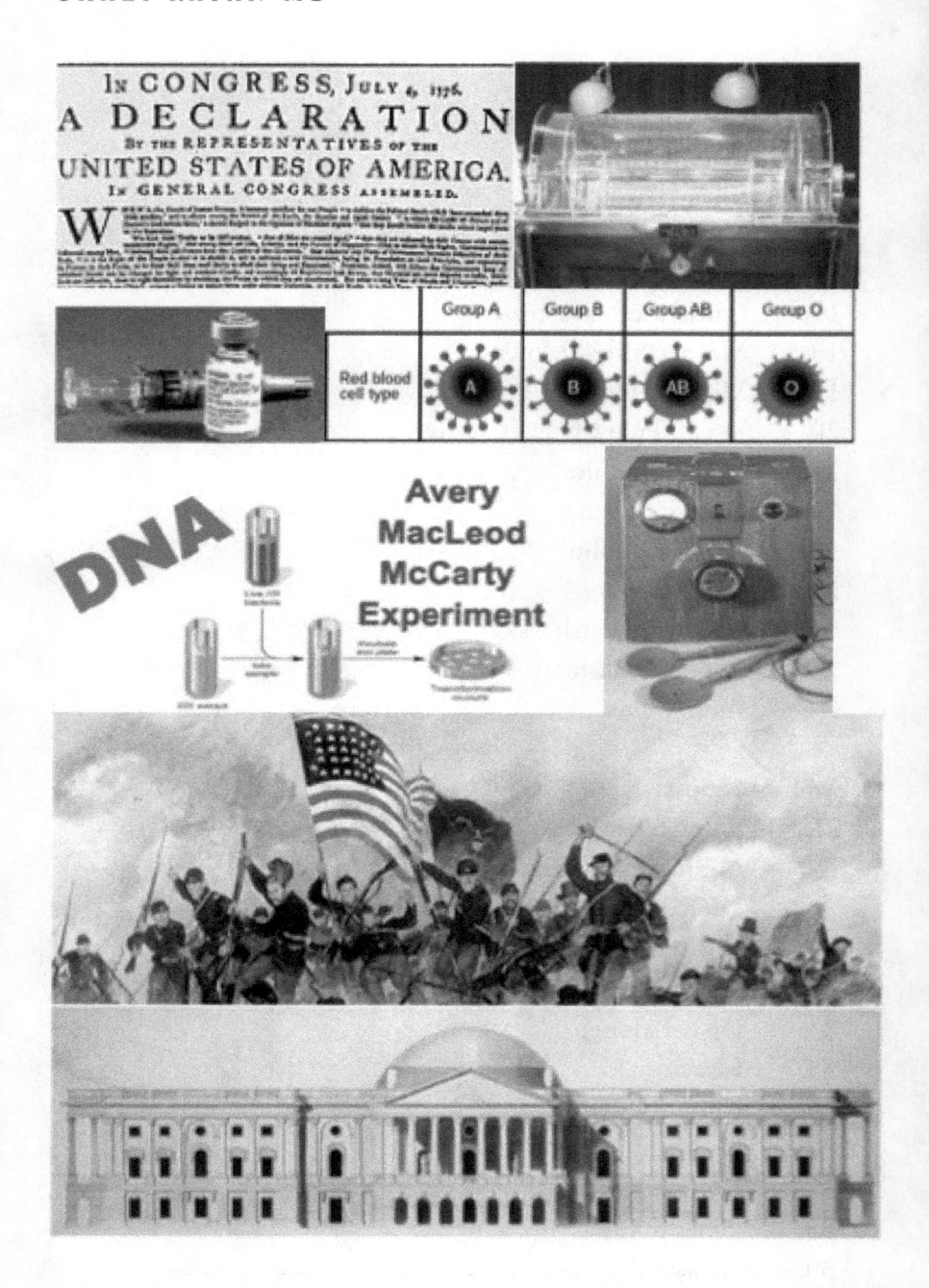

Gifts and inventions by immigrant physicians

The following is a summary of some advancements, contributions and leading roles immigrant physicians played in shaping medical history, aiding American Healthcare and laying the foundation of modern medicine:

Served as the earliest anatomy professors in American universities and discovered novel anatomical structures in human body and described their functions.

Contributed to medical education, revamped medical school admissions, enhanced medical schools' teaching curricula and created the residency training programs for physicians.

Introduced Orthopedic Surgery, and Pediatrics as specialties in the US and founded new American medical organizations such Cardiology Gynecology and Neurology.

Advanced endocrinology discipline and hormone and antibiotics therapies.

Initiated lifesaving artificial respiration and formulated local anesthetic for surgery.

Built public bathhouses, schools for the blind, field ambulances, ship hospital and global medical centers.

Enhanced hygiene practices and sanitary conditions in many communities, eradicated certain diseases and controlled disease epidemics, and passed city ordinances and federal legislations that improved overall patients' health and hygiene.

Classified blood groups that allowed safe transfusion and described the process of blood formation or hematopoiesis.

Probed deep in the molecular structure of cells with electron microscopy, demystified DNA, and elucidated genes' makeup and function.

GHAZI RAYAN MD

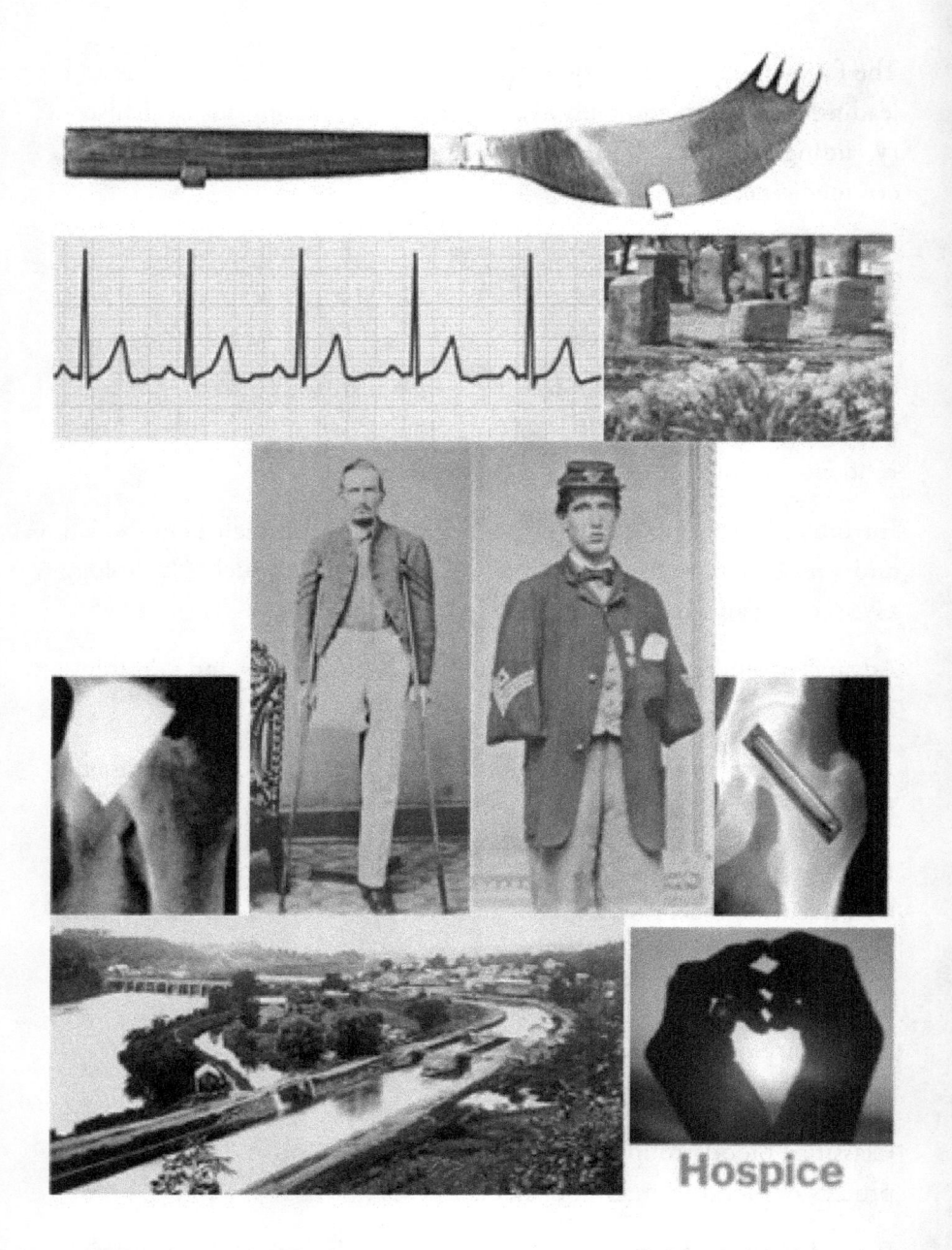

Gifts and inventions by immigrant physicians

Developed vaccines as for polio and tests that saved women's lives like Pap smear and men's lives by therapies for prostate cancer.

Perfected medical ultrasound techniques and made devices that helped rehabilitation of war veteran amputees.

Invented machines like kidney dialysis, heart catheters, cardiac defibrillator, EKG continuous recording and implantable heart.

Designed joint replacement and bone fixation devices and devised surgical methods to treat congenital and paralytic limb disorders.

Enriched the psychiatry discipline and refined Electro-Convulsive Therapy for treating psychiatric disorders.

Founded the study of healthcare quality and outcomes research.

Received Nobel and Pulitzer Prizes and Lasker awards for numerous medical research accomplishments.

Immigrant women physicians supported the suffrage movement, paved the way for other women's medical education, built medical schools for their gender, advanced obstetrical anesthesia and pediatric care, prevented catastrophic birth defects among newborn children and introduced hospice system and spread its services.

Immigrant physicians served as religious leaders during the colonial times; delegates to the Continental Congresses and Constitutional Convention during the Independence; patriots and military leaders during the Revolutionary War; gifted their lives on the battlefields during the Civil war; became politicians and state senators and governors during antebellum. They also made non-medical contributions such as proposing Ere Canal construction; architectural design of US State Capitol; making ink for printing money; inventing certain telescopes and astronomical instruments and developing cooling and early refrigeration systems.

Acknowledgments

My gratitude goes to Stanley Hupfeld and Bruce Lawrence previous CEOs at Oklahoma Integris Health for reviewing American Healthcare chapter. Managing at the same organization my daughter Nadine informs me of Hospital Systems Operations. I am thankful to Charles Bethea MD for his feedback about immigrant cardiologists and history of cardiology. My colleague and guide Roy Meals MD has been always willing to offer advice since I was his junior orthopedic resident in Baltimore Maryland. I am appreciative to Andy Sullivan MD and William Herndon MD for some information about orthopedic surgery history. Search engines such as Wikipedia the online encyclopedia and Google were indispensable for generating preliminary information and initial listings of many immigrant physicians essential to the topic of this book. Similarly Wikipedia and Library of Congress were godsend for trove of public domain images of immigrant physicians some of which were included in this book. The Metropolitan Library system of Oklahoma City was a great source for lending out myriad books that allowed me to delve deep into the detailed lives of immigrants and history of medicine. The Oklahoma Historical Society and Full Circle Bookstore in Oklahoma City have been supportive by sponsoring book signings and educational events. Thanks also go to Pamela Schroeder from the American Society for Surgery of the Hand for membership information and my deep appreciation goes to Alexandra Lapointe and Jack Joseph from Palmetto Publishing for their help, patience and support. Ultimately, we are all indebted to the early Immigrant American physicians mentioned in this book, and to many others, who came before and after them, but lost to history, for their medical triumphs and benefitting mankind; they were the inspiration for me writing this book. And then finally, and perhaps most importantly, my adoration goes to my adopted country America who opened its welcoming arms of inclusivity and offered opportunities to many immigrants like myself.

About the Author

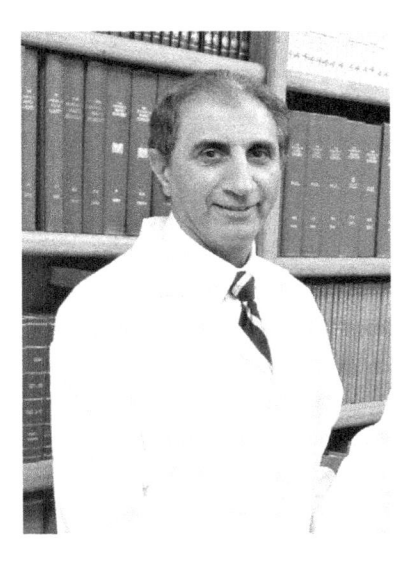

Ghazi Rayan is a first-generation immigrant American, a clinical professor of orthopedic surgery, and practiced as an orthopedic upper extremity hand surgeon in Oklahoma City. He established the first hand surgery fellowship in Oklahoma. Ghazi devoted most of his professional career serving his community, providing remedial care to his patients along with offering scientific knowledge in the form of research and teaching to medical students, residents and fellows. He is past president of the American Society for Surgery of the Hand and the recipient of several honors and awards.

Ghazi gave over 300, regional, national and inter-national scientific presentations. He is the author of nine academic books, and written over 40 book chapters and more than 200 scientific articles and editorials in peer-reviewed journals. He coauthored nonfiction titled *Trilogy of Perseverance and Friendship in the Golden Years* and his last nonfiction was *Immigrants who Founded and Fostered an Early Nation* (2021).

Ghazi and his wife live in Oklahoma City and relish the company of their three grandchildren. He continues serving his community and devoted to biking, reading and writing. More about Ghazi's background and journey through medicine are chronicled in the last chapter of this book.

Printed in the USA
CPSIA information can be obtained
at www.ICGtesting.com
LVHW091347270724
786433LV00002B/8